Study Guide to Accompar.

PSYCHIATRIC MENTAL HEALTH NURSING

4th Edition

Study Guide to Accompany

PSYCHIATRIC MENTAL HEALTH NURSING

4th Edition

Noreen Cavan Frisch, RN, PhD, FAAN
Professor and Chair
Department of Nursing
Cleveland State University
Cleveland, Ohio

Lawrence E. Frisch, MPH, PhD
Department of Preventive Medicine
The University of Kansas School of Medicine—Wichita
Wichita, Kansas

Prepared by
Linda B. Hureston, RN, PhD, CNE
Chicago State University
Chicago, Illinois

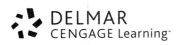
DELMAR
CENGAGE Learning™

Australia • Brazil • Japan • Korea • Mexico • Singapore • Spain • United Kingdom • United States

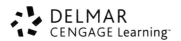

DELMAR
CENGAGE Learning

Study Guide to Accompany Psychiatric Mental Health Nursing
4th Edition

By Noreen Cavan Frisch and Lawrence E. Frisch

Vice President, Career and Professional Editorial:
Dave Garza

Director of Learning Solutions: Matt Kane

Senior Acquisitions Editor: Maureen Rosener

Managing Editor: Marah Bellegarde

Senior Product Manager: Juliet Steiner

Editorial Assistant: Samantha Miller

Vice President, Career and Professional Marketing:
Jennifer Ann Baker

Executive Marketing Manager: Wendy Mapstone

Senior Marketing Manager: Michele McTighe

Marketing Coordinator: Scott Chrysler

Production Director: Carolyn Miller

Production Manager: Andrew Crouth

Senior Content Project Manager: Stacey Lamodi

Senior Art Director: Jack Pendleton

For product information and technology assistance, contact us at
Professional & Career Group Customer Support 1-800-648-7450

For permission to use material from this text or product,
submit all requests online at **www.cengage.com/permissions**.
Further permissions questions can be e-mailed to
permissionrequest@cengage.com

Library of Congress Control Number: 2009925005

ISBN-13: 978-1-4354-0079-5
ISBN-10: 1-4354-0079-8

Delmar
5 Maxwell Drive
Clifton Park, NY 12065-2919
USA

Cengage Learning is a leading provider of customized learning solutions with office locations around the globe, including Singapore, the United Kingdom, Australia, Mexico, Brazil, and Japan. Locate your local office at:
international.cengage.com/region

Cengage Learning products are represented in Canada by Nelson Education, Ltd.

To learn more about Delmar, visit **www.cengage.com/delmar**

Purchase any of our products at your local college store or at our preferred online store **www.cengagebrain.com**

Notice to the Reader

Publisher does not warrant or guarantee any of the products described herein or perform any independent analysis in connection with any of the product information contained herein. Publisher does not assume, and expressly disclaims, any obligation to obtain and include information other than that provided to it by the manufacturer. The reader is expressly warned to consider and adopt all safety precautions that might be indicated by the activities described herein and to avoid all potential hazards. By following the instructions contained herein, the reader willingly assumes all risks in connection with such instructions. The publisher makes no representations or warranties of any kind, including but not limited to, the warranties of fitness for particular purpose or merchantability, nor are any such representations implied with respect to the material set forth herein, and the publisher takes no responsibility with respect to such material. The publisher shall not be liable for any special, consequential, or exemplary damages resulting, in whole or part, from the readers' use of, or reliance upon, this material.

Printed in the United States of America
1 2 3 4 5 6 7 14 13 12 11 10

Contents

UNIT III: SPECIAL POPULATIONS

UNIT IV: NURSING INTERVENTIONS AND TREATMENT MODALITIES

UNIT V: ADDITIONAL RESOURCES

Preface

The purpose of the *Study Guide to Accompany Psychiatric Mental Health Nursing* is to help you learn, absorb, and retain difficult and often unfamiliar concepts in psychiatric nursing. Although this *Study Guide* will not serve as a substitute for reading *Psychiatric Mental Health Nursing*, it will help reinforce the major concepts as you review the central facts of each chapter and suggest study strategies that will help you retain the material, perform well on tests, and develop the psychiatric knowledge and skills you will need to succeed as a nurse in any health care setting.

Each chapter of the *Study Guide* covers three areas: key terms, exercises and activities, and self-assessment.

Key Terms

The language of psychiatric nursing is specialized and sometimes difficult. Avoid the temptation to skip over this element in the textbook and in the *Study Guide*. Learning how to use this potent and interesting language will enhance your performance in the course and increase your effectiveness as a nurse. As a nurse, you need to be able to explain these concepts to your clients and their families, and you need to use these terms correctly and easily in your communication with your colleagues and other health professionals. The best time to learn terminology is the first time you encounter it.

Exercises and Activities

The Exercises and Activities sections identify the key concepts in the textbook chapters and challenge you to relate the concepts of psychiatric nursing to your own life and experience. There is no better teacher than your own experience. If you can relate the textbook content to your own life, to people you have known, even to movies and television shows you have seen and to books you have read, the knowledge will be personal and meaningful to you.

Self-Assessment Quizzes

If you can answer the test questions in the self-test correctly and confidently, then you have mastered most of the essential content of these chapters. The Self-Assessment Quizzes offer a great way to test your knowledge strengths and weaknesses.

The combination of *Psychiatric Mental Health Nursing* and this *Study Guide*, along with your clinical exposure, your instructor, and your classmates, should make this course in psychiatric nursing an intensely personal and rewarding experience for you. Psychiatric nursing may or may not have been what attracted you to nursing in the first place. However, it is our hope that what you gain from this experience will enhance your effectiveness as a nurse in ways you could never have imagined before this term began.

Chapter 1

THROUGH THE DOOR: YOUR FIRST DAY IN PSYCHIATRIC NURSING

The purpose of this chapter is to explore your own feelings and attitudes toward psychiatric mental health nursing. The chapter offers strategies for coping in the strange new world of psychiatric nursing. It helps you anticipate some of the role changes and rites of passage ahead of you in this course.

READING ASSIGNMENT

Please read Chapter 1, "Through the Door: Your First Day in Psychiatric Nursing," pages 2-13.

KEY TERMS

Write definitions for the following terms in your own words. Compare your definitions with those given in the text.

Depression _____

_____

Disability_____

_____

Distress _____

_____

Hallucination _____

_____

Mania _____

_____

Mental Disorder _____

_____

Mental Health_____

_____

Mental Illness _____

_____

Psychosis _____

_____

EXERCISES AND ACTIVITIES

1. Read the chapter opening on page 2. Answer the following questions in your own words.

   a. What has been your experience with and exposure to psychiatric nursing?

   _____

   _____

   _____

   _____

   _____

   b. What are your ideas and images of psychiatry and mental health care? Where do they come from?

   _____

   _____

   _____

   _____

   _____

   c. What are your feelings about taking a course in psychiatric mental health nursing? Are you anxious? Interested? Curious?

   _____

   _____

   _____

   _____

   _____

d. Mentally ill people are often stigmatized. What negative beliefs does the public hold for mentally ill people? Do you share any of these beliefs?

_____

_____

_____

_____

_____

2. Brainstorm a list of your own personality traits and personal characteristics. Arrange them in two columns labeled *Mentally Healthy* and *Mentally Unhealthy.*

Mentally Healthy	Mentally Unhealthy
_____	_____
_____	_____
_____	_____
_____	_____
_____	_____

Take a critical look at the results. Are you satisfied with the balance?

_____

_____

_____

_____

_____

3. Read "The Parallel Universe," by Susanna Kaysen, on pages 6–7.

a. Is "parallel universe" a good analogy for mental illness? Why or why not?

_____

_____

_____

_____

_____

b. What does the author mean by "Every window on Alcatraz has a view of San Francisco"?

_____

_____

_____

_____

_____

4. Read the Nursing Tip 1-1 on page 9.

a. What should your main focus be when starting a conversation with a psychotic client?

_____

_____

_____

_____

_____

b. List some ways you can build rapport with a psychotic client; include both verbal and nonverbal strategies.

_____

_____

_____

_____

c. The authors emphasize the importance of "listening, watching, and being there." What do they mean by "being there"? How might a depressed client respond to your "being there"? Can you think of other nonpsychiatric nursing experiences you've had when "being there" was therapeutic?

_____

_____

_____

_____

_____

5. Read "Student Nurses" on page 10.

a. Does the client's perception and opinion of student nurses surprise you?

_____

_____

_____

_____

_____

b. How do her responses compare to the responses of other clients you have met in nonpsychiatric settings?

_____

_____

_____

_____

6. Start a journal and keep it throughout the course. You might consider writing about certain themes that you can follow through this once-in-a-lifetime learning experience; for example, how your attitude toward mentally ill individuals evolves over time. Also, are there concepts and behaviors you just don't understand? How is your role changing? Will you become more confident of your skills? Who are some of the memorable clients and staff members you have met? What insights will you gain that will make you a better nurse, even in a regular medical setting?

7. Read the Advice from Prior Students on page 10. Log on to the Frisch Online Companion (http://www.delmarlearning.com/companions/). Based on your experience, offer your advice to future students of psychiatric mental health nursing.

8. Try repeating the following affirmations to yourself:

    "I can tolerate a certain amount of ambiguity."

    "Don't be afraid to make a mistake."

    "Mistakes are opportunities to learn."

    "I can trust the staff to look out for me."

    "People respond most positively to me when I am just myself."

    Write some affirmations that are tailored to meet your specific needs as you begin your study of psychiatric mental health nursing.

    _____

    _____

    _____

    _____

    _____

SELF-ASSESSMENT QUIZ

1. *Psychosis* means that an individual (page 7)

    a. suffers from mental retardation.

    b. has lost the ability to recognize reality.

    c. experiences bouts of alcoholism.

    d. is visually impaired.

2. People who are profoundly *depressed* (page 7)

    a. display boundless energy.

    b. talk in a boring monotone.

    c. may need to be protected against suicidal impulses.

    d. need rest and relaxation.

3. *Mania* is manifested by which of the following traits? (page 7)

    a. Remarkable memory

    b. Smiles and gestures

    c. Poutiness

    d. Exaggerated sense of well-being

4. A client on the psychiatric unit approaches the nursing students and states, "The voices are telling me to kick one of you." The students would interpret the client's statement as which of the following? (page 7)

    a. An hallucination

    b. A delusion

    c. Active depression

    d. Acute mania

5. The nurse manager of a psychiatric unit approaches a group of nursing students and begins discussing their new psychiatric rotation. When asked by the students, "What is mental illness?" the nurse manager would correctly respond by saying that the American Psychological Association (APA) defines mental illness as (page 6)

    a. the existence of poor health practices and outcomes resulting from major life stressors or traumatic experiences.

    b. the absence of positive mental health with potential of being harmful to self and/or others, or inability to care for self or personal finances.

    c. clinically significant behavior or psychological syndrome or pattern that occurs in an individual and is associated with present distress or disability.

    d. any situation, actual or perceived, requiring the development of newly structured adaptive coping mechanisms or professional intervention.

6. Although some students wish they didn't have to take psychiatric mental health nursing, the authors suggest benefits every nursing student might derive from this course. These benefits include which of the following? (pages 4, 9, 10)

    a. Discovering you might want to become a psychiatric nurse

    b. Mastering interpersonal skills essential in any nursing setting

    c. Gaining new insights into yourself that will make you a better nurse

    d. All of the above

7. One of the major factors that will facilitate student success in a psychiatric nursing course would include which of the following? (page 10)

   a. Shadowing an experienced RN for at least a day

   b. Taking time to reflect on how he or she comes across to others

   c. Assessing all of the client's weaknesses during the first encounter

   d. Discouraging clients from sharing feelings that may cause the client or student to become upset

8. A nursing instructor asks her student about the role of the RN on a psychiatric unit. The instructors would evaluate that a student understands if the student responds with which of the following statements? (page 8)

   a. "The RN provides recreation, diversional activity aimed at increasing socialization and activity."

   b. "The RN manages the impatient nursing care of clients; administers medications; completes assessments on clients; establishes outcomes; writes nursing diagnoses; and implements a plan of care that includes client/family teaching."

   c. "The RN provides psychotherapy; prescribes psychotropic medications (in most states); and manages and coordinates client care."

   d. "The RN manages patient care; admits patients to the hospital; prescribes psychotropic medications; and provides in-depth psychotherapy."

9. The most important nursing strategy that a nursing student will use when caring for a client with mental illness is (page 5)

   a. the ability to complete charting on time.

   b. communicating effectively with clients.

   c. avoiding upsetting the clients and staff.

   d. sharing personal experiences with a client.

10. A nursing instructor will evaluate that a student understands mental illness if the student states (page 5)

   a. "Mentally ill people are legally insane but they can't help being that way."

   b. "People who are mentally ill should always be placed on a locked unit."

   c. "A person can have symptoms of mental illness without being mentally ill."

   d. "I don't understand why we need to take this course; all we do is talk to people."

11. A nursing student asks the instructor, "Why are these clients on an acute psychiatric unit and not being seen in the clinic?" The most appropriate response by the instructor would be which of the following statements? (page 7)

    a. "I'm not sure but you can probably find out if you check with the charge nurse."

    b. "The client's insurance will cover hospitalization but not visits to a mental health clinic."

    c. "Clients on an acute psychiatric unit are there because they are ill and in need of supervision."

    d. "All clients with symptoms of mental illness need to be confined from the rest of society so they won't hurt anyone."

12. Define *rites of passage.* (page 4)

    _____

    _____

    _____

    _____

    _____

13. What do you think the authors mean by the phrase "being present"? (page 6)

    _____

    _____

    _____

    _____

    _____

Chapter 2

PSYCHIATRIC NURSING: EVOLUTION OF A SPECIALTY

The purpose of Chapter 2 is to build a context for how psychiatric nursing developed and why it is needed. Along the way, the chapter identifies some of the pioneers of psychiatric nursing and the major legislation that has led to the modern treatment of mental illnesses.

READING ASSIGNMENT

Please read Chapter 2, "Psychiatric Nursing: Evolution of a Specialty," pages 14–25.

KEY TERMS

Write definitions for the following terms in your own words. Compare your definitions with those given in the text.

Asylum _____

_____

Brown Report _____

_____

National Mental Health Act _____

_____

Psychiatric Mental Health Advanced Practice Registered Nurse _____

_____

Psychiatric Mental Health Nurse _____

_____

EXERCISES AND ACTIVITIES

1. Read the chapter opening on page 14. Compare and contrast psychiatric nursing with other nursing specialties.

   _____

   _____

   _____

   _____

   _____

2. Read Reflective Thinking 2-1 on page 17.

   a. Who do you think the "deviants" are in our current society?

   _____

   _____

   _____

   _____

   _____

   b. What does the contemporary treatment of mentally ill people say about our society and our values?

   _____

   _____

   _____

   _____

   _____

3. Study Van Gogh's painting on page 18.

   a. What characteristics of the care of the mentally ill in the nineteenth century are depicted in this painting?

   _____

   _____

   _____

   _____

   _____

   b. What observations can you make about the communication taking place in this painting? In what ways would communication be different in a mental health setting today?

   _____

   _____

   _____

   _____

   _____

4. The following events are referenced in Table 2-2 on page 21. To develop a sense of how psychiatric nursing has evolved over the past two centuries, match the year with the important event that took place that year:

   _____The National League for Nursing made psychiatric nursing a requirement for accreditation of basic nursing programs.

   _____Publication of the first psychiatric nursing textbook, *Nursing Mental Diseases*, by Harriet Bailey.

   _____Publication of *Interpersonal Relations in Nursing* by nurse theorist Hildegard Peplau.

   _____First mental hospital in the United States established in Williamsburg, Virginia.

   _____Publication of the Brown Report, which recommended that psychiatric nursing be included in general nursing education.

   _____First use of the term *psychiatry* by physicians attempting to upgrade the status of their work with the mentally ill.

_____Johns Hopkins Hospital included psychiatric nursing in the course of study for general nurses.

_____First school for psychiatric nurses (or mental nurses) established at the McLean Asylum in Somerville, Massachusetts.

_____Passage of the National Mental Health Act, which established the National Institutes of Mental Health (NIMH).

Check your answers in the text.

5. Create a timeline of important events in the history and practice of psychiatric mental health nursing. Update it throughout the course.

6. Review Table 2-1 on page 17, summarizing theories of mental illness formulated in the nineteenth century. Based on what you know today, what would you call our current understanding of mental illness, and what are its premises? Do you expect your view to evolve during this course?

_____

_____

_____

_____

_____

7. Briefly summarize the contributions of these pioneers of psychiatric nursing:

a. Dorothea Lynde Dix

_____

_____

_____

_____

_____

b. Isabel Hampton Robb

_____

_____

_____

_____

_____

c. Lavinia Lloyd Dock

_____

_____

_____

_____

_____

8. List as many career opportunities for the psychiatric nurse, outside of a locked psychiatric hospital, as you can.

_____

_____

_____

_____

_____

9. Characterize the challenge of the future of psychiatric nursing.

_____

_____

_____

_____

_____

SELF-ASSESSMENT QUIZ

1. Of the following, which is not an important publication in the history of psychiatric nursing? (page 21)

    a. *Utilitarianism* by John Stuart Mill

    b. *Nursing Mental Diseases* by Harriet Bailey

    c. *Interpersonal Relations in Nursing* by Hildegard Peplau

    d. *The Brown Report* by Esther Lucille Brown

2. Nursing training schools were established at leading psychiatric hospitals because (page 18)

    a. the asylums wanted free labor.

    b. there was a need to recruit women to care for people with mental illnesses.

    c. there weren't enough doctors to take care of all the clients.

    d. the Civil War had produced an abundance of mentally ill people.

3. According to McCabe (2005), which of the following disorders is the leading cause of disability? (page 22)

    a. Schizophrenia

    b. Major depressive disorders

    c. Personality disorders

    d. Dissociative disorders

4. According to McCabe (2005), psychiatric disorders account for what percentage of the burden of disease in the United States? (page 22)

    a. 15%

    b. 20%

    c. 32%

    d. 45%

5. The degeneracy theory of mental illness focused on which of the following beliefs? (page 17)

    a. Belief that infection causes insanity

    b. Belief that those who are ill can contaminate others

    c. Belief that persons are mentally ill by virtue of having bad character

    d. Belief that dirt and putrefaction are the principal causes of illness

6. *Nursing Mental Diseases* was which of the following? (page 21)

    a. The first psychiatric nursing textbook published

    b. A report of the results of a five-year project funded by the NIMH

    c. The first theoretical framework for the practice of psychiatric nursing

    d. An article written by Lucille Brown and published in the *American Journal of Nursing*

7. According to the American Nurses Association (ANA) standards, the preparation for certification at the basic level of practice is the (page 21)

    a. CAN.

    b. LPN.

    c. RN.

    d. APRN.

8. Match the time period in the left-hand column to the prevalence of the treatment modalities in the right-hand column. (pages 16–20)

    _____Ancient times   a. Isolation from society

    _____Middle Ages   b. Reverence or repulsion

    _____Late 1800s   c. Insulin and electric shock

    _____Early 1900s   d. Physical labor

    _____1920s   e. Hot and cold packs

    _____1930s   f. Psychopharmacology

    _____1950s   g. Humane custodial care

9. Match the psychiatric pioneer with his or her unique contribution. (pages 17–20)

____Hildegard Peplau   a. Early believer in treating mental illness as disease

____Dorothea Dix   b. Early advocate of training for nurses

____William Battie   c. First required psychiatric nursing in nursing curriculum

____Edward Cowles   d. Started formal training for mental health nurses

____Isabel Hampton Robb   e. Advocated affiliation between nursing schools and
                                    psychiatric hospitals
____Effie Taylor
                                f. Defined nurse-client relationships
____Esther Brown
                                g. Advocated humane treatment of the mentally ill

Chapter 3

THEORY AS A BASIS FOR PRACTICE

The purpose of Chapter 3 is to establish the theoretical basis of psychiatric nursing. After first discussing theories specific to nursing, the chapter discusses the major theories of psychology.

READING ASSIGNMENT

Please read Chapter 3, "Theory as a Basis for Practice," pages 26–58.

KEY TERMS

Write definitions for the following terms in your own words. Compare your definitions with those in the text.

Adaptive Potential _____

_____

Choice Point _____

_____

Cognator Subsystem _____

_____

Cognition _____

_____

Concept _____

_____

Conceptual Framework_____

_____

Created Environment _____

_____

Culture _____

_____

Culture Care _____

_____

Culture Care Accommodation/Negotiation _____

_____

Culture Care Preservation/Maintenance _____

_____

Culture Care Repatterning/Restructuring _____

_____

Ego _____

_____

External Environment _____

_____

Extrapersonal Stressor _____

_____

Fixation_____

_____

Generic or Folk Care Activities _____

_____

Helicy _____

_____

Id _____

_____

Integrality _____

_____

Internal Environment _____

_____

Interpersonal Stressor _____

_____

Intrapersonal Stressor _____

_____

Modeling_____

_____

Nursing Agency _____

_____

Nursing System _____

_____

Orientation Phase _____

_____

Professional Care-Cure Practices _____

_____

Regression _____

_____

Regulator Subsystem _____

_____

Resonancy _____

_____

Role-Modeling _____

_____

Self-Care _____

_____

Self-Care Agency_____

_____

Self-Care Deficit _____

_____

Superego _____

_____

Termination Phase _____

_____

Theory _____

_____

Therapeutic Self-Care Demand_____

_____

Working Phase   _____

_____

EXERCISES AND ACTIVITIES

1. Read the chapter opening on page 26.

    a   Write a definition for the word *theory*.

    _____

    _____

    b. How is the word *theory* used in everyday conversation?

    _____

    _____

    _____

    _____

    _____

    c. How is the word *theory* used in a discipline?

    _____

    _____

    _____

    _____

    _____

2. Review Reflective Thinking 3-1 concerning theory on page 30.

    a. Why is theory important to nursing practice?

_____

_____

_____

_____

_____

    b. Give examples of how your nursing practice might vary if you moved from one nursing theory to another. Think about a specific client care situation and ask yourself how your response might differ from theory to theory.

_____

_____

_____

_____

_____

3. Explain the differences between a *theory,* a *concept,* and a *conceptual framework.* Which is the most general idea? Give an example of each.

_____

_____

_____

_____

_____

4. Name the three stages of the nurse's relationship with the client in Peplau's Interpersonal Relations in Nursing Theory, discussed on page 30. Do you agree that this is a regular pattern in your relationship to your clients? Can you think of examples from your own experience that followed this pattern?

_____

_____

_____

_____

_____

5. The authors identify four general classes of nursing theories:

1. Theories based on relationships

2. Theories based on caring

3. Theories based on energy fields

4. Theories based on when nursing is needed

   a. Match the classes of theories with the theorists below by identifying which class of theories applies to each theorist: (pages 30-41)

   _____Leininger

   _____Parse

   _____Betty Neuman

   _____Roy

   _____Rogers

   _____Orem

   _____Margaret Newman

   _____Watson

   _____Peplau

   _____Boykin and Shoenhofer

   _____Erickson, Tomlin, and Swain

6. Identify the psychological theorists based on their identification of the ages and stages of man:

   a. _____Trust vs. mistrust; autonomy vs. shame and doubt; initiative vs. guilt; industry vs. inferiority; identity vs. role confusion; intimacy vs. isolation; generativity vs. stagnation; ego integrity vs. despair

   b. _____Sensorimotor intelligence; preoperational thought; concrete operations; formal operations

   c. _____Physiological needs; safety and security; love and belonging; esteem and self-esteem; self-actualization

   d. _____Oral stage; anal stage; phallic stage; latency age; puberty

7. Explain how nursing theories and psychological theories can work together. Do nursing theories account for human development and explain mental illness? Do psychological theories offer guidance on nursing practice?

   _____

   _____

   _____

   _____

   _____

8. Jean Watson's model of Intentional Transpersonal Human Caring has recently been updated. Please answer the following questions about it:

   a. Characterize the difference between curing and caring.

   _____

   _____

   _____

   _____

   _____

b. Define *intentionality*.

c. Do you cultivate your spiritual self each day? If so, what do you do? If not, what actions could you take to do so?

9. What similarities do you see between Orem's nursing theory and existential philosophy?

10. Review Reflective Thinking 3-5 about sociocultural perspective on page 54.

a. List the nursing theories you think reflect a more sociocultural perspective.

b. List those that tend to view the individual in isolation of his or her sociocultural surroundings.

_____

_____

_____

_____

_____

c. Divide the psychological development theories in like manner.

_____

_____

_____

_____

_____

d. Do you see any similarities between the nursing theories and psychological theories that place people in a sociocultural context?

_____

_____

_____

_____

_____

e. Do you see any similarities between the nursing theory and psychological theories that attempt to understand individuals apart from their contextual surroundings?

_____

_____

_____

_____

_____

11.	Read Reflective Thinking 3-6 on page 54 about the "myth" of mental illness. Considering that definitions and responses to mental illness throughout history have changed and evolved, is it possible that our current conception of mental illness is wrong? Is the current view of mental illness just a reflection of the twentieth century's obsession with science, rationality, and medical advances? How would you refute Szasz's arguments?

_____

_____

_____

_____

_____

SELF-ASSESSMENT QUIZ

1.	Hildegard Peplau's nursing theory is based on therapeutic _____. (pages 30-31)

2.	The key concept associated with Erickson, Tomlin, and Swain's nursing theory is _____. (pages 31-32)

3.	Two nursing theories based on caring were developed by _____ and _____. (pages 32-34)

4.	Rogers, Parse, and Newman developed nursing theories based on _____ _____. (pages 35-38)

5.	Orem's theory is known as _____ _____ _____. (page 38)

6.	Freud identified three aspects of the personality, which he termed _____, _____, and _____. (pages 41, 43-45)

7.	The psychological theorist most closely associated with the ages and stages of man is _____. (pages 45-47)

8.	Harry Stack Sullivan believed that people grow psychologically in the context of their _____ relationships. (pages 47-48)

9. Piaget is associated with the _____ development of children. (pages 48-49)

10. Skinner is classified as a _____ psychologist. (pages 52-53)

11. To a nurse who bases her practice on theory, which of the following is not an advantage? (page 29)

    a. Being able to more easily transfer knowledge and experience from one situation to another

    b. Being able to communicate about nursing practice to others

    c. Being able to judge appropriateness of behavior in specific circumstances

    d. Being able to practice on the same plane as physicians and pharmacists

12. Sociocultural Theory holds that (page 54)

    a. there is no such thing as mental illness.

    b. society may be "sicker" than its individuals.

    c. culture, society, government, laws, regions, and the economy can all contribute to mental illness.

    d. government programs can be designed to prevent or lessen the severity of mental illness.

13. Which of the following form the building blocks of theory? (page 29)

    a. Concepts

    b. Frameworks

    c. Hypotheses

    d. Paradigms

14. Which theorist tried to show that humans behave in much the same way as pigeons and rats? (page 50)

    a. Freud

    b. Piaget

    c. Skinner

    d. Sullivan

15. The psychiatric nurse establishes nursing interventions that are based on a caring philosophy. The nurse's approach to care is most likely influenced by the work of which of the following nurse theorists? (page 32)

    a. Jean Watson

    b. Callista Roy

    c. Dorothea Orem

    d. Hildegard Peplau

16. A 21-year-old college student is seen in the campus health center after being raped. The nurse would recognize that the student is in which stage of Erikson's theory of growth and development? (page 46)

    a. Trust versus mistrust

    b. Intimacy versus isolation

    c. Identity versus role confusion

    d. Ego integrity versus despair

17. While conducting a session with a client, the client states, "I feel so guilty about what I did." The nurse understands that the client's guilt is based on which component of Freud's theory of personality development? (page 43)

    a. Id

    b. Ego

    c. Superego

    d. Libido

Chapter 4

NEUROSCIENCE AS A BASIS FOR PRACTICE

The purpose of Chapter 4 is to establish the theoretical basis of psychiatric nursing. This chapter discusses the contemporary view of the biological basis of mental illness. It may seem odd at first to think of consciousness, emotions, and thoughts in terms of biological processes going on in the nervous and regulatory systems. However, in this chapter, we explore the methodology and findings associated with the relationship between neuroscience and behavior.

READING ASSIGNMENT

Please read Chapter 4, "Neuroscience as a Basis for Practice," pages 60–77.

KEY TERMS

Write definitions for the following terms in your own words. Compare your definitions with those given in the text.

Computerized Tomography (CT) _____

_____

Cortex _____

_____

Deoxyribonucleic Acid (DNA) _____

_____

Diencephalon _____

_____

Genetic Marker _____

_____

Genome _____

_____

Hypothalamus _____

_____

Magnetic Resonance Imaging (MRI) _____

_____

Neurotransmitter _____

_____

Positron Emission Tomography (PET) _____

_____

Synapse_____

_____

Thalamus _____

_____

EXERCISES AND ACTIVITIES

1. Refer to the discussion of brain anatomy in Figure 4-1 on page 63.

    a. What are the four main divisions of the central nervous system?

        _____

        _____

        _____

        _____

    b. Which of these is related to consciousness and psychiatric disorders?

        _____

    c. Identify the importance, in terms of behavior, of the thalamus and the hypothalamus.

        _____

        _____

        _____

        _____

        _____

d. Identify the four lobes of the cortex, and explain their functions and significance.

_____

_____

_____

_____

_____

2. Define *biopsychophysiological theory.* (page 62)

_____

_____

_____

_____

a. How is this theory different from the "classic" theories of psychology and their explanations of mental illness?

_____

_____

_____

_____

b. What similarities and differences do you see between Skinner's behavioral theory and the biopsychophysiological theory?

_____

_____

_____

_____

3. The hypothalamus controls the autonomic nervous system. Explain how it regulates changes in our bodies when we experience anxiety. (page 64)

_____

_____

_____

_____

_____

4. Identify the three major brain-imaging technologies and briefly describe the unique advantages of each. (pages 65–67)

_____

_____

_____

_____

_____

5. Study the material on electrophysiology and neurochemistry on pages 67–71.

   a. Label the structures of the microanatomy of a neuron, reproduced below.

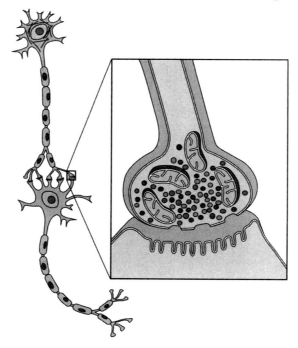

b. State the sequence of events that nerve cells undergo in the process of passing information from one cell to the next.

_____

_____

_____

_____

_____

c. Did the discussion of electrophysiology give you any additional insights into the "energy field" nursing theories discussed in the beginning of this chapter? What are they?

_____

_____

_____

_____

_____

6. Study the section on neurotransmitters on page 69–70.

a. What characterizes substances as neurotransmitters?

_____

_____

_____

_____

b. Describe the basic mechanism of all neurotransmitters.

_____

_____

_____

_____

c. What is the difference between excitatory stimulation and inhibitory stimulation?

_____

_____

_____

_____

_____

d. How do neurons "know" whether to fire their own action potentials in the presence of numerous neurotransmitters?

_____

_____

_____

_____

_____

7. What recent discovery about membrane receptors explains why clozapine, unlike typical neuroleptic drugs, blocks delusions and hallucinations without causing side effects that resemble Parkinson's disease? (page 71)

_____

_____

_____

_____

8. What is the relationship between DNA, RNA, and proteins that comprise amino acids? (pages 71–72)

_____

_____

_____

_____

9. What is the significance of mapping the human genome for the understanding and treatment of mental illness? (page 73)

_____

_____

_____

_____

10. What is meant by the term *blood oxygen dependent contrast*? (page 66)

_____

_____

_____

SELF-ASSESSMENT QUIZ

1. Biopsychophysiology involves the study of all of the following except (page 62)
   a. biochemistry.
   b. genetics.
   c. neuroanatomy.
   d. anthropology.

2. The diencephalon includes (page 64)
   a. the thyroid and the thalamus.
   b. the thyroid and the parathyroid.
   c. the thalamus and the hypothalamus.
   d. the hypothalamus and the pituitary.

3. Structures in the brain connected with the production of memories and emotions include (page 65)
   a. the limbic system, the amygdala, the hypothalamus, and the cortex.
   b. the limbic system, the amygdala, the hypothalamus, and the optic nerve.
   c. the limbic system, the auditory nerve, the hypothalamus, and the cortex.
   d. the amygdala, the hypothalamus, the cortex, and the optic nerve.

4. Which of the following is not an imaging technology? (pages 65–67)

    a. Computerized tomography

    b. Magnetic resonance imaging

    c. Primal scream therapy

    d. Positron emission tomography

5. Name the four lobes of the cortex. (page 64)

    a. Prefrontal, frontal, parietal, and occipital

    b. Frontal, temporal, spatial, and parietal

    c. Frontal, temporal, occipital, and parietal

    d. Frontal, temporal, occular, and precipital

6. Which of the following statements about synapses is not correct? (page 69)

    a. Synapses are very wide compared to gap junctions.

    b. The mechanisms of transmission across synapses are much less complex than those governing transmission across gap junctions.

    c. Ions don't flow across synapses.

    d. Most psychiatric medications act upon the nerve synapses.

7. Which of the following statements about neurotransmitters is not correct?

    a. Neurotransmitters either excite or inhibit a dentrite.

    b. Neurotransmitters don't cross synaptic clefts.

    c. Neurotransmitters can be controlled precisely by reuptake into the axon that released them.

    d. Many psychiatric drugs prevent the reuptake of neurotransmitters.

8. During the first few weeks of life, memory storage is the function of which aspect of the brain? (page 65)

    a. Limbic system

    b. Cerebellum

    c. Spinal cord

    d. Frontal lobe

9. Which of the following scanning techniques allows scientists to determine which neurotransmitters and chemicals are present at specific brain sites? (page 67)

    a. Magnetic resonance imaging (MRI)

    b. Magnetic resonance spectroscopy (MRS)

    c. Diffusion tensor imaging (DTI)

    d. Positron emission tomography (PET)

10. Recent studies have found that in addition to peptides, another set of brain chemicals modifies the way in which synapses respond to electrical stimulation. These chemicals are known as (page 71)

    a. alcobinoids.

    b. cannabinoids.

    c. neurobinoids.

    d. peptobinoids.

11. Which of the following scanning techniques allows brain white fibers to be visualized? (page 67)

    a. Magnetic resonance imaging (MRI)

    b. Magnetic resonance spectroscopy (MRS)

    c. Diffusion tensor imaging (DTI)

    d. Positron emission tomography (PET)

12. Which of the following best describes the human genome? (page 72)

    a. The entire complex of heritable information

    b. A highly variable molecule that consists of two strands

    c. Identifiable patterns of DNA structure

    d. Cells to which a neurotransmitter combines

Chapter 5

DIAGNOSTIC SYSTEMS FOR PSYCHIATRIC NURSING

The purpose of this chapter is to explain the various systems for labeling and classifying mental disorders, from both a medical and a nursing standpoint, showing how medical and nursing systems interact. The purposes of these systems are explained, and issues like privacy, confidentiality, and communications among health professionals are explored.

READING ASSIGNMENT

Please read Chapter 5, "Diagnostic Systems for Psychiatric Nursing," pages 78–96.

KEY TERMS

Write definitions for the following terms in your own words. Compare your definitions with those given in the text.

Classification _____

_____

DSM-IV-TR _____

_____

HIPAA _____

_____

ICD _____

_____

ICNP _____

_____

NANDA _____

_____

NIC _____

_____

NMDS _____

SNOMED _____

UMLS _____

EXERCISES AND ACTIVITIES

1. Prior to reading this chapter, how familiar were you with the language and systems of psychiatric nursing? Have you used some of these terms before? Were you using the language correctly? Write down areas in which the chapter clarified, corrected, or sharpened your previous knowledge of this specialized language.

    _____

    _____

    _____

    _____

    _____

2. Describe the purpose of each of the following diagnostic systems: (pages 81–89)

    a. DSM _____

    _____

    b. ICD _____

    _____

    c. NANDA _____

    _____

3. Read Case Example 5-1, "Maria," on page 81.

    a. Would you know which classification system to use when caring for Maria?

    _____

b. Would you use more than one classification system? Which ones, and why?

_____

_____

_____

_____

_____

4. Review Box 5-1, "DSM Axial Diagnoses for Case 5-1: Maria," on page 84.

a. Do you agree with the diagnoses, based on the information given?

_____

b. Explain why "recent divorce" would be included under Axis IV.

_____

_____

_____

_____

_____

5. Review Table 5-1, "Global Assessment of Functioning Scale," on page 83.

a. Do you agree with the score of 60 assigned to Maria in the case example? Why or why not?

_____

_____

_____

_____

_____

b. Rate another client you have recently encountered, using the GAF Scale. Explain the rationale for your assessment.

_____

_____

_____

_____

_____

c. Would you find this scale useful in your nursing experience? List the advantages and the drawbacks as you see them.

_____

_____

_____

_____

_____

6. Review Nursing Alert 5-1, "Cultural Sensitivity and DSM," on page 84.

a. Explain why cultural issues might be important to consider before arriving at a psychiatric diagnosis.

_____

_____

_____

_____

_____

b. Do you believe that, ultimately, diagnostic criteria transcend cultural differences? Why or why not?

_____

_____

_____

_____

_____

7. Explain why the American Psychiatric Association updated the DSM to DSM-IV-TR in 2000. How would you characterize the changes?

_____

_____

_____

_____

_____

8. Review Reflective Thinking 5-1, "Pros and Cons of a Psychiatric Diagnostic System," on page 85.

    a. Do you think a psychiatric center could function effectively without diagnostic systems? How would it function differently if there were no psychiatric diagnostic systems?

    _____

    _____

    _____

    _____

    _____

    b. Respond to the following statement: "A nurse should be able to respond therapeutically to a client's behavior without having to categorize or label a client with a diagnosis."

    _____

    _____

    _____

    _____

    _____

9. Review Reflective Thinking 5-2, "What Is Unnamed Is Unnoticed," on page 86.

    a. How would you respond to a client who displays the following symptoms?

        Self-esteem disturbance

        _____
        _____
        _____
        _____
        _____

        Powerlessness

        _____
        _____
        _____
        _____
        _____

        Sleep pattern disturbance

        _____
        _____
        _____
        _____
        _____

    b. What strategies would you use to interact with this client?

        _____
        _____
        _____
        _____
        _____

c. Provide a sample documentation of the client's diagnosis and your interventions.

_____

_____

_____

_____

_____

10. Read Reflective Thinking 5-3, "Are Nursing Diagnoses Useful?" on page 89.

a. In your own words, state your attitude toward nursing diagnoses.

_____

_____

_____

_____

_____

b. How are you expected to use nursing diagnoses in this course?

_____

_____

_____

_____

_____

c. State the rationale for the way nursing diagnoses are used in this course, and comment on their professional value.

_____

_____

_____

_____

_____

11. Review Table 5-2, "Diagnoses from Three Systems for Case Example: Maria," on page 90.

    a. Which of these diagnoses is most useful to you in planning your nursing care?

_____

_____

_____

_____

_____

    b. Do any of these diagnoses give you so little information that you can't use them in planning nursing care?

_____

12. Review the discussion of the Health Insurance Portability and Accountability Act of 1996 (HIPAA), on page 92.

    a. What are the provisions and requirement of the Act?

_____

_____

_____

_____

_____

    b. What are the drawbacks and loopholes of the Act?

_____

_____

_____

_____

_____

c. How do you expect HIPAA to affect the nursing profession?

_____

_____

_____

_____

_____

13. Read the material on pages 93–94 related to recent advances in diagnostic nomenclature.

a. Write out the full meanings of these acronyms:

UMLS _____

_____

SNOMED _____

_____

NMDS _____

_____

ICNP _____

_____

b. What implications would these advances have for your daily nursing practice?

_____

_____

_____

_____

_____

14. Obtain a copy of the journal *Nursing Diagnosis* and review the articles and issues discussed. What relevance do the issues in this journal have to the way you want to practice nursing?

_____

_____

_____

_____

_____

15. Explain how the Nursing Outcomes Classification (NOC) is structured. (page 91)

_____

_____

_____

_____

_____

SELF-ASSESSMENT QUIZ

1. The nurse planning client care would refer to which classification system to identify clinical tasks or activities that can be carried out by the nurse to assist in the client's treatment? (page 90)

   a. NANDA-I

   b. DSM-IV-TR

   c. NIC

   d. NOC

2. When assessing a client, the nurse would most likely refer to which classification system to identify a specific psychiatric disorder? (page 82)

   a. NANDA-I

   b. DSM-IV-TR

   c. NIC

   d. NOC

3. Which classification system would the nurse find most useful when establishing outcomes for client care? (page 91)

    a. NANDA-I

    b. DSM-IV-TR

    c. NIC

    d. NOC

4. A nurse assigned to the emergency department would find which document most useful when identifying an appropriate nursing diagnosis reflective of the assessed data? (page 85)

    a. NANDA-I

    b. DSM-IV-TR

    c. NIC

    d. NOC

5. A client is admitted with a diagnosis of hypochondriasis. The nurse would find this diagnosis on which axis of the DSM-IV-TR? (page 82)

    a. Axis I

    b. Axis II

    c. Axis III

    d. Axis IV

Chapter 6

TOOLS OF PSYCHIATRIC MENTAL HEALTH NURSING: COMMUNICATION, NURSING PROCESS, AND THE NURSE-CLIENT RELATIONSHIP

The purpose of this chapter is to develop the tools and skills set necessary to function effectively as a psychiatric nurse. Many of these skills are psychosocial interactive skills you will find transfer readily to any nursing setting as well as to the care of nonpsychiatric clients.

READING ASSIGNMENT

Please read Chapter 6, "Tools of Psychiatric Mental Health Nursing: Communication, Nursing Process, and the Nurse-Client Relationship," pages 98–117.

KEY TERMS

Write definitions for the following terms in your own words. Compare your definitions with those given in the text.

Concept Map _____

_____

Defense Mechanisms _____

_____

Feedback _____

_____

Nonverbal Communication _____

_____

Nursing Care Plan _____

_____

Orientation Phase _____

_____

Process Recording _____

_____

Termination Phase _____

_____

Therapeutic Communication _____

_____

Working Phase _____

_____

EXERCISES AND ACTIVITIES

1. Read the chapter opening on page 98.

   a. What are some of the techniques you could use in establishing therapeutic relationships with clients?

   _____

   _____

   _____

   _____

   _____

   b. Identify the characteristics and differences between a therapeutic relationship and a personal relationship.

   _____

   _____

   _____

   _____

   _____

2. Review Reflective Thinking 6-1 on page 102. List your most characteristic nonverbal gestures. Think about your smile, eye contact, hand movements, head nodding, and eyebrow movements.

_____

_____

_____

_____

_____

3. Review Reflective Thinking 6-2 on page 102. Under what circumstances would you consider "invading" a client's space, and why might this action be therapeutic in effect?

_____

_____

_____

_____

_____

4. Study the "Summary of Therapeutic Communication Techniques" in Table 6-1 on page 104.

   a. Test yourself by covering one column at a time and filling in the missing content.

   b. Restate the meaning of each technique in your own words, including the purpose of each.

_____

_____

_____

_____

_____

_____

_____

_____

_____

_____

5. Review Table 6-2, "Common Defense Mechanisms," on page 105.

    a. Test yourself by covering one column at a time and filling in the missing content.

    b. In the following spaces, write an example for each of the defense mechanisms drawn from your own recent clinical experience. If you can't think of an example for one or more, ask your classmates or instructor to suggest an example.

        Symbolization

        _____

        Sublimation

        _____

        Suppression

        _____

        Regression

        _____

        Reaction formation

        _____

        Displacement

        _____

        Introjection

        _____

        Rationalization

        _____

        Repression

        _____

        Projection

        _____

        Denial

        _____

6. Read the "Sample Process Recording" in Table 6-3 on page 106.

    a. Write a process recording drawn from a recent therapeutic interaction you have had with a client. Structure and analyze it according to the format in Table 6-3.

    b. Critique your example. Is there anything you would have changed about the interaction?

_____

_____

_____

_____

_____

7. Review Figure 6-2, "Two Views of the Nursing Process," on page 107. Which view appeals more to you? Why?

_____

_____

_____

_____

_____

8. Review Table 6-4, "Elements of a Psychiatric History," on page 108. Note that the last item in the table is "Critical Decisions." Identify which of the preceding items in the table might contribute to the critical decisions, and explain why.

_____

_____

_____

_____

_____

9. Review Table 6-5 on page 109 and think about the nursing process.

   a. Explain the relationship between the elements of a psychiatric history (Table 6-4, page 108) and the nursing assessment.

_____

_____

_____

_____

_____

10. Explain the difference between a nursing care plan and a care map, noting the advantages of each. (You may want to study a completed care map such as the one in Chapter 11, pages 202–204.) Which do you prefer? Which does your instructor prefer?

_____

_____

_____

_____

_____

11. Write a nursing care plan for a client you have worked with recently. Convert it to a concept map.

12. Explain how you selected the nursing diagnosis in your plan. Would you need to have a therapeutic relationship with the client to accurately select the nursing diagnosis?

_____

_____

_____

_____

_____

13. Review Box 6-1, "Five Aims of Intervention," on page 111. Do the interventions in your care plan address all five aims? Why or why not?

_____

_____

_____

_____

_____

14. Read Case Example 6-1, "Mrs. Rose M," on page 114.

    a. In your own words, describe the phases of the nurse-client relationship as it is used in this case example.

_____

_____

_____

_____

_____

    b. Which steps of the nursing process seem to correlate with each phase of the nurse-client interaction relationship?

_____

_____

_____

_____

_____

SELF-ASSESSMENT QUIZ

1. "Unconscious responses used by individuals to protect themselves from internal conflict and external stress" is a definition for which of the following terms? (pages 104–105)

    a. Reflection

    b. Nonverbal communication

    c. Paralinguistic cues

    d. Defense mechanisms

2. All of the following are examples of nonverbal communication except (pages 101–103)

    a. physical space.

    b. action or kinetics.

    c. touch.

    d. listening.

3. When a nursing student does a process recording, he or she should (page 106)

    a. tape record the conversation with the client and listen to it with the class.

    b. take notes during the conversation and take it to the supervisor for interpretation.

    c. write a nearly verbatim account of the conversation with the client, and interpret the techniques used and their effectiveness.

    d. write a report summarizing the conversation and use it to help formulate a nursing care plan.

4. Therapeutic communication techniques are best described as (page 105)

    a. listening, silence, and suggesting.

    b. broad openings, restating, and informing.

    c. clarification, reflection, focusing, and confronting.

    d. all of the above.

5. The nursing process incorporates which of the following elements? (page 107)

    a. Critical decision making, mental status examination, past medical history, and chief complaint

    b. Identifying data, developmental and psychosocial history, outcomes, and present illness history

    c. Mental status examination, planning interventions, nursing diagnosis, and outcomes

    d. Assessment, nursing diagnosis, planning interventions, and evaluation

6. Which of the following are examples of defense mechanisms? (page 105)

    a. Symbolization and denial

    b. Projection and displacement

    c. Regression and relating

    d. a and b

    e. a and c

7. All of the following are elements of a psychiatric history except (page 108)

    a. critical decisions.

    b. identifying data.

    c. impaired social interaction.

    d. mental status examination.

8. Nursing diagnoses frequently seen in psychiatric nursing include all the following except (page 109)

    a. risk for injury.

    b. depression.

    c. social isolation.

    d. post-trauma response.

9. The nurse-client relationship includes which of the following phases? (pages 112-113)

    a. Building trust phase, working phase, and termination phase

    b. Orientation phase, promotion of strength phase, and termination phase

    c. Orientation phase, working phase, and termination phase

    d. All of the above

10. An advantage of a nursing care plan over a care map is that (pages 111-112)

    a. a nursing care plan makes it easy to document and compare the observed outcome with the anticipated outcome.

    b. a nursing care plan is more contextually based.

    c. a nursing care plan enables the nurse to grasp assessment data and nursing diagnoses more holistically.

    d. a nursing care plan makes it easier for the nurse to identify priorities for care.

11. A nursing student is very angry at the instructor because the student failed several quizzes and received a failing grade on the process recording. However, the student brings the instructor a cup of coffee and a Danish each morning of class. The student's behavior is an example of which defense mechanism? (page 105)

    a. Introjection

    b. Sublimation

    c. Suppression

    d. Reaction formation

12. A client is being seen by a psychiatric social worker. The nurse has a role to know and understand the goals the social worker has for the client's care and to support the goals in her interaction with the client. The nurse in this situation is functioning in which type of role? (page 110)

    a. Dependent

    b. Independent

    c. Collaborative

    d. Submissive

13. The nurse is developing a care plan for a client who is feeling depressed, alone, and isolated. An appropriate short-term goal would be which of the following? (page 109)

    a. The client will form a one-on-one relationship with the nurse such that the client will talk with the nurse for 30 minutes daily.

    b. The client will build relationships with others in his environment and will interact socially with others at least two times throughout the day by 3 months' time.

    c. Within 1 month, the client will interact in a social setting with another person at least twice per week.

    d. The client will be less isolated and more willing to participate in all unit activities.

14. During a conversation with a client, the client indicates she wants to find a new place to live. The nurse responds, "Are you saying you want to move out of your current apartment?" The nurse's response is an example of which therapeutic communication technique? (pages 103–104)

    a. Restating

    b. Focusing

    c. Clarification

    d. Confronting

15. For the past two individual sessions with the nurse therapist, a client discusses his experiences at school. Today in their meeting, the nurse states, "Let's go back to the situation at school where you felt uncomfortable in class." The nurse's statement is an example of which therapeutic communication technique? (pages 103–104)

    a. Restating

    b. Focusing

    c. Clarification

    d. Confronting

16. A student nurse tells her classmates that she failed the psych quiz even though she knew all of the material. She further states that the instructor had too many trick questions on the test. Which defense mechanism is the student most likely using? (page 105)

    a. Denial

    b. Projection

    c. Displacement

    d. Rationalization

Chapter 7

CULTURAL AND ETHNIC CONSIDERATIONS

The purpose of this chapter is to frame your thinking about the role of culture in mental illness and its treatment. This chapter encourages you to develop an awareness of your own culture and cultural identity, which can influence your feelings toward mental illness. You will consider the values and attitudes that act as prisms—coloring, refracting, distorting, and magnifying the cultural differences among individuals—as you encounter and treat people with mental illnesses.

READING ASSIGNMENT

Please read Chapter 7, "Cultural and Ethnic Considerations," pages 118–131.

KEY TERMS

Write definitions for the following terms in your own words. Compare your definitions with those given in the text.

Cultural Blindness _____

_____

Cultural Facilitator/Broker _____

_____

Culture _____

_____

Culture Shock_____

_____

Ethnicity _____

_____

Ethnocentrism _____

_____

Norms _____

_____

Stereotyping _____

_____

Values _____

_____

EXERCISES AND ACTIVITIES

1. Read the chapter opening on page 118. Describe what you think another person might perceive about your cultural identity and cultural beliefs.

   _____

   _____

   _____

   _____

   _____

2. On page 122, the authors state that many nursing models of cultural assessment have been developed, citing Giger and Davidhizar and Andrews and Boyle as examples. They then explain the model they have used to organize this chapter. Have you thought about how you organize your cultural assessments? Develop a model you could use in your own practice, using the models cited for guidance.

   _____

   _____

   _____

   _____

   _____

3. Besides Western biomedical causation, name five agents that people worldwide believe cause mental illness. (page 122)

_____

_____

_____

_____

_____

4. Read the section on Care Seeking and Acceptable Care on pages 123–124.

   a. List the factors you can think of that people use to avoid or delay seeking general medical care.

   _____

   _____

   _____

   _____

   _____

   _____

   b. List other factors that are roadblocks specific to seeking psychiatric mental health care.

   _____

   _____

   _____

   _____

   _____

   c. How would you counsel a person to overcome these particular reasons for not seeking psychiatric care?

   _____

   _____

   _____

   _____

   _____

5. Seek out a person with a cultural background different from your own and engage the person in a casual conversation, making note of the following: (pages 125–127)

a. Eye contact

_____

_____

b. Proxemics (space and time)

_____

_____

c. Touch

_____

_____

d. Silence

_____

_____

e. Social behavior

_____

_____

f. Time orientation

_____

_____

6. Read the section on Time Orientation on page 127.

    a. Are you sequentially oriented or synchronically oriented? Why? Give an example.

_____

_____

    b. How would you determine which time orientation another person has?

_____

_____

_____

_____

_____

    c. What strategies would you use to interact effectively with a person whose time orientation is the opposite of your own?

_____

_____

_____

_____

_____

7. Write your personal definition of a "culturally competent" mental health nurse. (pages 128–129)

_____

_____

_____

_____

_____

8. As a cultural experiment, begin a conversation with a friend who has the same cultural background as you do. During the conversation, move in close to your friend, closer than you feel would be normal. (page 126)

a. How uncomfortable did this feel, and how long did it take for the discomfort to develop? What was your friend's reaction?

_____

_____

_____

_____

_____

b. Repeat the experiment, using silence as the variable. How long did your friend tolerate the silence? How uncomfortable do you feel in being silent during a conversation with your friend?

_____

_____

_____

_____

_____

c. For people who may be depressed, anxious, or even psychotic, how much more uncomfortable do you think these violations of cultural norms would make them feel?

_____

_____

_____

_____

_____

9. Describe an incident in which you felt culturally out of place. Be sure to try to recreate your feelings. (pages 120–121)

_____

_____

_____

_____

_____

10. You may already be aware that pain thresholds vary widely among cultural groups. Identify two other biological differences among cultural groups that have significance for the care and treatment of mental illness. (pages 127–128)

_____

_____

_____

_____

_____

11. Discuss how you would demonstrate cultural sensitivity in your role as a psychiatric nurse.

_____

_____

_____

_____

_____

SELF-ASSESSMENT QUIZ

1. The nurse is scheduled to see a client who is always late for appointments. The nurse would recognize that punctuality is (page 127)

    a. related to a person's time orientation.

    b. a rare commodity that should be cherished.

    c. a concept with different meanings for clients with mental illness.

    d. always a sign of resistance to therapy.

2. The nurse who is culturally sensitive should (page 120)

    a. treat everyone the same and ignore differences in culture.

    b. provide the best care to individuals whose culture is the same as that of the nurse.

    c. recognize that one's own worldview is the only acceptable truth.

    d. make an effort to understand more about a client's culture in order to provide the best care.

3. In the mainstream American culture, time is often believed to be (page 127)

    a. equal to money.

    b. not very important.

    c. something to waste.

    d. a precious commodity.

4. Which of the following statements regarding cultural sensitivity is true? (pages 128–129)

    a. It is nice for nurses to be culturally sensitive, but it is not required.

    b. It is more important for psychiatric nurses to be culturally sensitive than nurses working in other specialties.

    c. Developing culturally sensitive practices can help reduce barriers to effective treatment utilization.

    d. Male nurses are more culturally sensitive than female nurses, and older nurses are more culturally sensitive than younger nurses.

5. The development of agranulocytosis is most common in which ethnic group? (pages 127–128)

    a. Arab Americans

    b. Jewish North Americans

    c. African Americans

    d. Asians/Pacific Islanders

6. All of the following can be barriers to cultural sensitivity except (pages 121–122)

    a. cultural encounters.

    b. ethnocentrism.

    c. stereotyping.

    d. cultural blindness.

7. Which of the following is a sure sign of mental illness? (pages 122–127)

    a. Abnormal behavior

    b. Inappropriate behavior

    c. Silence

    d. Rudeness

    e. None of the above

8. Mental illness can be attributed to (pages 122–123)

    a. sorcery.

    b. violating taboos.

    c. environmental imbalances.

    d. laziness.

9. A cultural facilitator or broker can do all of the following except (page 125)

    a. understand the health beliefs of the client's culture.

    b. arrange to pay for health care.

    c. interpret in the client's native language.

    d. explain the health care system to the client.

10. The communication problem a nurse can most easily solve is (page 128)

    a. unappreciated cultural considerations.

    b. altered thought processes.

    c. fear or mistrust.

    d. age and sex differences.

11. Match the term with the appropriate definition.

    ___ Norms

    ___ Values

    ___ Ethnocentrism

    ___ Cultural blindness

    ___ Ethnicity

    ___ Cultural sensitivity

    a. Learned beliefs about what is held to be good or bad in a culture

    b. The perception that our worldview is the only acceptable truth and that our beliefs, values, and sanctioned behaviors are superior to all others

    c. Learned behaviors that are perceived to be appropriate or inappropriate

    d. Expectation of all members of a particular culture to hold the same beliefs and behave in the same way

    e. An essential component in rendering effective culturally responsive care to all clients

    f. The attempt to treat all persons fairly by ignoring differences and acting as though the differences do not exist

Chapter 8

EPIDEMIOLOGY OF MENTAL HEALTH ILLNESS

The purpose of this chapter is to establish the incidence and prevalence of mental illness, to explain how mental illnesses are categorized and diagnosed, and to suggest research areas that need to be explored in future studies.

READING ASSIGNMENT

Please read Chapter 8, "Epidemiology of Mental Health Illness," pages 132–143.

KEY TERMS

Write definitions for the following terms in your own words. Compare your definitions with those given in the text.

Blinded Clinical Trial _____

_____

Case Control Study _____

_____

Cohort Study _____

_____

Control Group _____

_____

Controlled Clinical Trial_____

_____

Descriptive Study _____

_____

Double-Blinded Trial _____

_____

Endemic _____

_____

Epidemic_____

_____

Epidemiology _____

_____

Experimental Group _____

_____

Incidence _____

_____

Interrater Agreement _____

_____

Interrater Reliability _____

_____

Intrarater Reliability _____

_____

Longitudinal Study _____

_____

Meta-Analysis _____

_____

Placebo _____

_____

Prevalence _____

_____

Quasi-Experimental Study _____

_____

Reliability _____

_____

Risk Factors _____

_____

Validity _____

_____

EXERCISES AND ACTIVITIES

1. Read the chapter opening on page 132. What role do you feel nurses should play in the development of public health policy?

   _____

   _____

   _____

   _____

   _____

2. In your own words, state as many goals of epidemiology as you can. (pages 134–135)

   _____

   _____

   _____

   _____

   _____

3. Explain the difference between a blinded and a double-blinded controlled clinical trial. (page 135)

   _____

   _____

   _____

   _____

   _____

4. Explain the difference between incidence and prevalence. (page 136)

_____

_____

_____

_____

_____

5. Explain the difference between descriptive and quasi-experimental studies, and state the significance of the difference. (page 136)

_____

_____

_____

_____

_____

6. Take the timeline you created in Chapter 2 (Exercise and Activity #5) and superimpose the various revisions of the DSM on it. (pages 136–138)

   a. What correlations emerge?

   _____

   _____

   _____

   _____

   b. Add the major landmark studies referenced in this chapter, including the Epidemiologic Catchment Area Study.

   _____

   _____

   _____

   _____

7. In your own words, state the purposes of the DSM and its use in psychiatric nursing. (pages 136–137)

_____

_____

_____

_____

_____

8. Stigmatization is one of the major reasons why people with mental illnesses often avoid seeking treatment. Labeling contributes to stigmatizing. What devices do the authors of this textbook use to avoid labeling? Read Reflective Thinking 8-1 on page 137. What strategies can you incorporate into your own clinical practice to avoid labeling and unnecessary stigmatizing?

_____

_____

_____

_____

_____

9. Refer to the DSM-IV-TR Classification in Appendix A on page 931 for the currently accepted labels for the entire range of psychiatric disorders.

   a. Do any of these labels surprise you? Did this exercise enhance your understanding of the range of disorders classified as psychiatric disorders? Did this exercise help you organize mental disorders better in your mind?

   _____

   _____

   _____

   _____

   _____

b. Review the descriptions of mood disorders, schizophrenia, substance abuse
    disorders, and anxiety disorders on page 137. List the major diagnostic criteria for
    each of these groups of disorders.

Mood disorders

_____

_____

_____

_____

_____

Schizophrenia

_____

_____

_____

_____

_____

Substance abuse disorders

_____

_____

_____

_____

_____

Anxiety disorders

_____

_____

_____

_____

_____

c. How difficult do you think it would be to diagnose someone with one of these disorders?

_____

_____

_____

_____

_____

10. What were the significant findings of the three early epidemiological studies in Stirling County, Nova Scotia; Manhattan; and Baltimore? (page 138)

_____

_____

_____

_____

_____

11. Review the questions on page 138 raised by the Carter Commission. For which of these questions was the resulting Epidemiologic Catchment Area (ECA) Study able to provide some answers?

_____

_____

_____

_____

_____

12. Which results of the ECA Study surprised you the most? (page 139)

_____

_____

_____

_____

_____

13. What is the *tip-of-the-iceberg phenomenon?* (page 140)

_____

_____

_____

_____

_____

14. Summarize the main finding of the National Comorbidity Study (NCS). How would you compare the comorbidity of psychiatric disorders with that of medical-surgical disorders? (page 141)

_____

_____

_____

_____

_____

SELF-ASSESSMENT QUIZ

1. A nurse epidemiologist identifies that 25 new cases of a disease have been diagnosed in a community. The nurse understands that this number represents the (page 136)

   a. epidemiology.

   b. prevalence.

   c. incidence.

   d. pandemic.

2. A nurse epidemiologist identifies that there are a total of 100 residents of a community diagnosed with a particular disease. The nurse understands that this number represents the (page 136)

   a. epidemiology.

   b. prevalence.

   c. incidence.

   d. pandemic.

3. The ECA study found that which conditions were the most prevalent? (page 140)

    a. Depression and mania

    b. Schizophrenia and alcoholism

    c. Alcohol and substance abuse

    d. Dependent personality and hypochondriasis

4. An epidemiologic study where neither the subject nor the person evaluating the outcomes knows whether the subject is receiving active treatment or placebo is known as a (page 135)

    a. descriptive study.

    b. correlational study.

    c. case control study.

    d. double-blind trial.

5. Epidemiology allows nurse researchers to study (page 134)

    a. only diseases.

    b. only treatments.

    c. both diseases and treatments.

    d. neither diseases nor treatments.

6. The Carter Commission wanted answers to which of the following questions? (page 138)

    a. How much would a massive mental health study cost?

    b. Should Medicare cover major mental disorders?

    c. What are the causes of mental illness?

    d. Does poverty contribute to the severity of mental illness?

    e. b and c

    f. c and d

7. Which of the following is *not* a result of choosing the wrong sample size for a study? (page 139)

    a. People won't have confidence in the results if it is too small.

    b. The results won't be valid if it is too small.

    c. The results will be confusing if it is too big.

    d. A sample too large would be a waste of money.

8. The *tip-of-the-iceberg phenomenon* means that (page 140)

    a. many people have symptoms, but only a few seek help.

    b. only a small number of mentally ill people are severely mentally ill.

    c. life is fraught with hidden perils.

    d. there are not enough resources to care for everyone with mental illness.

9. According to the NCS, what is the comorbidity? (page 141)

    a. 10%

    b. 90%

    c. 70%

    d. 50%

10. Cognitive impairment is (page 139)

    a. not a DSM diagnosis.

    b. more prevalent among older people.

    c. a major, underrecognized public health problem.

    d. all of the above.

Chapter 9

ETHICAL AND LEGAL BASES FOR CARE

The purpose of this chapter is to provide you with the ethical theories and legal information you need to guide your practice. Conducting nursing care in a manner that conforms to the law and adheres to the highest ethical standards protects you from lawsuits and protects your clients from abuse, manipulation, and shoddy health care. In the area of mental health practice, there are many unique ethical issues and highly specific laws that apply to the conduct of psychiatric care.

READING ASSIGNMENT

Please read Chapter 9, "Ethical and Legal Bases for Care," pages 144–161.

KEY TERMS

Write definitions for the following terms in your own words. Compare your definitions with those given in the text.

Abandonment _____

_____

Autonomy _____

_____

Beneficence _____

_____

Civil Commitment _____

_____

Code of Ethics _____

_____

Competency to Stand Trial _____

_____

Conservator _____

_____

Deontology _____

_____

Emergency Hospitalization _____

_____

Ethics _____

_____

Fidelity _____

_____

Incompetence _____

_____

Justice _____

_____

Least Restrictive Alternative _____

_____

Malpractice _____

_____

M'Naghten Test _____

_____

Negligence _____

_____

Nonmaleficence _____

_____

Normative Ethics _____

_____

Physical Restraint _____

_____

Probate Proceedings _____

_____

Seclusion _____

_____

Tarasoff Duty to Warn _____

_____

Utilitarianism _____

_____

EXERCISES AND ACTIVITIES

1. Read the chapter opening on page 144.

   a. Do you feel in control when you have a client under your care? List ways in which you have power or control over that client.

   _____

   _____

   _____

   _____

   _____

   b. Do you conduct your professional practice in a manner deserving of the trust the public has in the nursing profession? List some of the "rules" you have that guide your practice.

   _____

   _____

   _____

   _____

   _____

2. Read Reflective Thinking 9-1 on page 147.

    a. Do you think Harold needs health care help? What would you do to try to help him?

_____

_____

_____

_____

_____

    b. Would you enlist the support of any other health care professionals to help him?

_____

_____

_____

_____

_____

3. Write your response to the authors' observation that "laws attempt to provide for the public good and public safety, but rarely do the laws offer comprehensive solutions to social problems." (page 150)

_____

_____

_____

_____

_____

4. Rules associated with the Health Insurance Portability and Accountability Act (HIPAA) went into effect in 2003. (page 151)

    a. Briefly summarize your obligations to keep patient information confidential.

    _____

    _____

    _____

    _____

    _____

    b. Explain when your obligation to keep patient information private is negated by other ethical and legal obligations you have.

    _____

    _____

    _____

    _____

    _____

5. Laws often regulate conflicting interests. Match the conflicting rights in the two columns by drawing lines between them. (pages 150–155)

Right to treatment	Right to safety
Right to an orderly treatment environment	Right of many against few
	Right to refuse treatment
Right to informed consent	Right not to be restrained or secluded
Right of free speech	
Right to privacy	Right to refuse consent
Right to keep personal items	Right to be informed of threats

6. What does the American Psychological Association's Mental Health Patient's Bill of Rights cover? What other rights, if any, do you think mental health patients should have? (pages 150-155)

_____

_____

_____

_____

_____

7. Mark David Chapman shot and killed John Lennon. Refusing the insanity defense, he pleaded guilty and received a sentence of 20 years to life. John Hinckley shot and wounded then-President Ronald Reagan in an effort to impress actress Jody Foster. He was found guilty by reason of insanity. The American poet Ezra Pound made radio broadcasts during World War II in support of Italian dictator Benito Mussolini and was charged with treason. He was kept in a psychiatric hospital for years before charges were dropped, and he was allowed to spend his remaining years in Italy. Juries rejected the insanity defense for serial killers Jeffrey Dahmer, John Wayne Gacy, and David "Son of Sam" Berkowitz (who later admitted he made up his story of receiving messages to kill from barking dogs). (page 153)

   a. What is the rule of law that provides for the insanity defense?

   _____

   _____

   _____

   _____

   _____

   b. What is your opinion of the insanity defense?

   _____

   _____

   _____

   _____

   _____

c. Could you provide quality nursing care for a client who had committed a crime but had been declared not guilty by reason of insanity?

_____

_____

_____

_____

_____

d. Ethically and/or legally, would you be under any obligation to provide treatment to that client?

_____

_____

_____

_____

_____

8. A widely cited New York case, *Rivers v. Katz* (1986), provides guidelines to determine when clients can be given medication against their will. (pages 153–155)

a. State the four guidelines established by the court.

_____

_____

_____

_____

_____

b. Are these guidelines used in your state? If not, are any other guidelines in place?

_____

_____

_____

_____

_____

9. Consider Reflective Thinking 9-5 on informed consent, regarding Mrs. Roebuck, on page 156.

    a. Is there a clear-cut consent to treatment from Mrs. Roebuck? Why or why not?

    _____

    _____

    _____

    _____

    _____

    b. If you were the nurse caring for Mrs. Roebuck, what would you do to make yourself feel more comfortable that the informed consent issue was handled properly?

    _____

    _____

    _____

    _____

    _____

10. What elements are necessary and desirable in obtaining informed consent? (page 153)

    _____

    _____

    _____

    _____

    _____

11. In dealing with clients who may have altered thought processes, extreme preoccupation, a flat affect, or regressed behavior, obtaining informed consent for treatment becomes a gray area of judgment for the clinician. (pages 153–155)

a. How would you decide whether a client had the capacity to provide informed consent?

_____

_____

_____

_____

_____

b. Are there any special measures you could take to demonstrate that informed consent was obtained in a careful, responsible manner?

_____

_____

_____

_____

_____

12. Numerous legal and ethical obligations apply to the psychiatric mental health nurse. Although laws vary from state to state, some well-established guidelines are virtually universal. (pages 157–159)

a. When a clinician becomes aware that a client has made a specific threat of bodily harm against a specific individual, what is the clinician's responsibility?

_____

_____

_____

_____

_____

b. When a clinician is informed that child abuse is taking place, what is the clinician's duty?

_____

_____

_____

_____

_____

c. When clinicians discontinue professional practice, what is their obligation to their clients?

_____

_____

_____

_____

_____

d. When is it appropriate for a clinician to have a sexual relationship with a client or former client?

_____

_____

_____

_____

_____

e. When is it appropriate to release confidential information about a client?

_____

_____

_____

_____

_____

f. When is it appropriate to violate the civil rights of a client?

_____

_____

_____

_____

_____

SELF-ASSESSMENT QUIZ

1. A client tells a nurse that he hates his doctor and plans to hurt the doctor. When the nurse returns to work the next day, she finds that the physician has been brutally beaten by the client and the physician is hospitalized. The nurse can be charged with which of the following? (page 157)

   a. Felony

   b. Malpractice

   c. Negligence

   d. Misdemeanor

2. When a health care provider does not inform an individual of a client's threat, the health care provider has ignored which of the following? (page 157)

   a. Tarasoff Duty to Warn

   b. Patient's Bill of Rights

   c. Community Mental Health Centers Act

   d. Rule of habeas corpus

3. The fundamental responsibilities of nurses are to (page 148)

   a. describe disease etiology, treat disease, and provide referrals.

   b. promote health, facilitate healing, and alleviate suffering.

   c. plan strategies, reflect on practice, and implement research.

   d. provide support, conduct research, and treat disease.

4. A nurse refuses to continue treating a client.This is an example of which of the following? (page 157)

   a. Burnout

   b. Abandonment

   c. Disenfranchisement

   d. Intolerance

5. The nurse's primary responsibility is to the (page 148)

   a. client.

   b. family.

   c. physician.

   d. employing agency.

6. All of the following are legitimate ethical theories used to guide ethical decision making in the health care sector except (page 147)

   a. situational ethics.

   b. utilitarianism.

   c. justice.

   d. autonomy.

7. Clients have all of the following rights except (pages 150–155)

   a. civil rights.

   b. the right to keep personal items.

   c. the right to choose the nurse assigned to them.

   d. the right to informed consent.

8. All of the following are the usual and prudent elements of informed consent except (page 153)

   a. all risks associated with the treatment.

   b. the description, length, and cost of treatment.

   c. a clinician's note in the client record and a consent signed by the client.

   d. the most significant risks associated with treatment.

9. For a client to be involuntarily committed to a psychiatric facility, a court has to hear compelling evidence of any of the following except that the client is (pages 155–156)

    a. dangerous to self.

    b. dangerous to others.

    c. insulting or vulgar to the judge.

    d. unable to care for basic needs.

10. The nurse has the right to release confidential information about a client in all but which one of the following situations? (page 151)

    a. The client signs a release.

    b. The client is a celebrity and the request comes from the media.

    c. An officer of the court has a signed court order.

    d. Another health professional is directly involved in the care of the client.

Chapter 10

SELF-CARE FOR THE NURSE

T he purpose of this chapter is to help you develop knowledge and techniques designed to reduce the stress of caring for clients with psychiatric disorders. Not surprisingly, many of the techniques and modalities that nurses use to reduce stress in clients can be used in self-care to prevent burnout, protect one's own health, and open up new horizons and opportunities in the practice of nursing.

READING ASSIGNMENT

Please read Chapter 10, "Self-Care for the Nurse," pages 162–178.

KEY TERMS

Write definitions for the following terms in your own words. Compare your definitions with those given in the text.

Burnout _____

_____

Circadian Rhythm _____

_____

Nurse-Self Care _____

_____

Parasympathetic System Response _____

_____

Sympathetic System Response _____

_____

EXERCISES AND ACTIVITIES

1. Have you ever watched a movie and left the theater feeling as if you had the power and charisma of the film's heroine or hero? Have you ever felt energized in the presence of a vivacious, charismatic, enthusiastic, elated, or cheerful person? (pages 164–165) Do you believe it is possible for you to create such positive feelings in a client through the personal magnetic power of your own presence? Can you give any examples of these phenomena?

   _____

   _____

   _____

   _____

   _____

2. The authors reference several books written by nurses that document their attraction to nursing and the odysseys they have taken in pursuing their careers. (pages 164–165) Have you read any other books by either nurses or clients that document their stories, aspirations, or struggles to achieve peacefulness, contentment, and reward in their lives?

   _____

   _____

   _____

   _____

   _____

3. Make a list of factors you think can contribute to nurse burnout. (page 165)

   _____

   _____

   _____

   _____

   _____

4. What does the acronym "HALT" stand for? Give an example of how you might use this technique as an internal self-assessment. (page 167)

_____

_____

_____

_____

_____

5. Name the six modalities nurses can use to refresh their physical, emotional, mental, and spiritual health and enhance their stamina and nursing performance. (pages 168–174)

_____

_____

_____

_____

_____

6. How do the forces associated with burnout affect your energy field? (page 165)

_____

_____

_____

_____

   a. How can you restore health to the energy field that surrounds you?

   _____

   _____

   _____

   _____

b. How can your clients benefit from a healthy vibrant energy field radiating from your physical presence?

_____

_____

_____

_____

_____

7. Activities like centering may seem "far out" or unscientific, and many nurses are skeptical about trying this technique. However, agree to suspend your judgment and practice centering, described on pages 171–172, for a full day the next time you are in a clinical setting. Then, record the results of your experiment here.

_____

_____

_____

_____

_____

8. Form a support group with some peers where you can practice the kinds of support interventions you all agree are most helpful. Ban griping and designate someone to be the "energy monitor." (page 174) What interventions are most effective?

_____

_____

9. With a group of your peers, listen to and discuss a motivational audiotape like Napoleon Hill's *Think and Grow Rich*. (page 174) Which strategies do you find to be most motivational?

_____

_____

10. Interview your peers to try to learn at least three new self-care techniques or insights today. (page 175) List the three techniques you think are best here.

_____

_____

_____

SELF-ASSESSMENT QUIZ

1. A nurse who evaluates her own energy field is most likely using the theory of which of the following nurse theorists? (page 172)

    a. Jean Watson

    b. Dorothea Orem

    c. Margaret Newman

    d. Martha Rogers

2. According to Rogers, nurses can calm the disturbing energy around them by (page 172)

    a. changing the client's energy field.

    b. changing their own energy field.

    c. actively participating in hospital governance.

    d. changing the environment of the work unit.

3. Optimal attentiveness usually lasts how many minutes? (page 167)

    a. 15–30 minutes

    b. 45–75 minutes

    c. 90–120 minutes

    d. 130–160 minutes

4. All of the following are self-help modalities except (pages 168–175)

    a. meditation.

    b. imagery.

    c. medication.

    d. self-hypnosis.

5. Recent studies have found which of the following? (pages 164–165)

   a. Nurses' worklives are becoming more difficult as patient acuity levels increase.

   b. Nurses' worklives are becoming less difficult as patient acuity levels increase.

   c. Nurses' worklives are becoming more difficult as patient acuity levels decrease.

   d. Nurses' worklives are not affected by patient acuity levels.

6. The personal benefits of imagery include all of the following except (pages 168–169)

   a. the benefits can be had within one minute, in any location.

   b. it can allow nurses to reconnect to their inner resources.

   c. it isolates nurses from their colleagues and clients.

   d. it can restore a sense of health and balance.

7. Techniques that facilitate meditation and deep relaxation include all of the following except (pages 169–170)

   a. any repetitive task as it can be conducive to meditation if the individual accepts the task as a joy in itself.

   b. breathing exercises.

   c. visualizing the peaceful inner workings of your healthy body.

   d. reviewing past injustices you have suffered.

8. A positive outcome of meditative self-care or self-hypnosis might be that (page 169)

   a. you can get by on less sleep if you meditate.

   b. you don't need to seek medical attention for a health problem if you try to heal yourself with your own mind.

   c. you can let your subconscious do your thinking for you.

   d. you might open your mind to new solutions to old problems.

9. All of the following are essential to centering except (pages 171–172)

   a. standing with squared shoulders, your feet firmly planted about twelve inches apart.

   b. releasing tension by taking several deep breaths and exhaling completely.

   c. feeling the earth beneath you supporting you and restoring your energy field.

   d. choosing to be fully present with your client, asking for spiritual guidance if necessary.

10. Positive physiological responses to laughter include all of the following except (pages 172-174)

    a. releasing endorphins, giving us a sense of control and mastery of our circumstances.

    b. improving the immune system, eliminating cancerous cells, and promoting the release of neurotransmitters.

    c. helping mask uncomfortable or painful feelings.

    d. dampening corticosteroid production, avoiding immunosuppression.

Chapter 11

THE CLIENT UNDERGOING CRISIS

The purpose of this chapter is to help you understand the stages of a crisis, evaluate coping mechanisms, and implement interventions that may lessen the impact of a crisis.

READING ASSIGNMENT

Please read Chapter 11, "The Client Undergoing Crisis," pages 180–207.

KEY TERMS

Write definitions for the following terms in your own words. Compare your definitions with those given in the text.

Adaptive Energy _____

_____

Adaptive Potential Assessment Model _____

_____

Arousal _____

_____

Community Crisis _____

_____

Conservative-Withdrawal State _____

_____

Crisis _____

_____

Cultural Crisis _____

_____

Culture Shock_____

_____

Equilibrium_____

_____

Fight-Flight Response _____

_____

General Adaptation Syndrome _____

_____

Impoverishment _____

_____

Maturational Crisis_____

_____

Psychological Development _____

_____

Situational Crisis _____

_____

Stress _____

_____

EXERCISES AND ACTIVITIES

1. Pick a crisis from your own experience and use it as a focal point throughout this chapter. (pages 183–184)

   a. Describe the crisis you've chosen. What type of crisis is it?

   _____

   _____

   _____

   _____

   _____

b. What support systems, if any, did you use in managing your crisis?

_____

_____

_____

_____

_____

c. What coping skills did you use to reduce your anxiety?

_____

_____

_____

_____

_____

d. What features of your personality did you use to help you cope with this crisis?

_____

_____

_____

_____

_____

e. What nursing theory would you suggest for a nurse caring for you in this crisis?

_____

_____

_____

_____

_____

2. Name and differentiate the four types of crises, noting their distinguishing characteristics. (page 184)

_____

_____

_____

_____

_____

3. What are Caplan's four phases of a crisis? (page 184)

_____

_____

_____

_____

_____

a. What can an individual do to escape from an escalating crisis?

_____

_____

_____

_____

_____

b. What possible outcomes can individuals experience if they are not able to prevent the escalation of a crisis?

_____

_____

_____

_____

_____

4. In response to their experience of the 9-11 crisis, the New York State Nurses Association asked the American Nurses Association to provide leadership and guidance for nurses dealing with such crises. List some of the measures you feel the ANA should pursue.

_____

_____

_____

_____

_____

5. What are the phases of Selye's General Adaptation Syndrome? Relate these phases to the personal crisis you identified above. What specific behaviors did you exhibit during the various phases of your crisis? (page 185)

_____

_____

_____

_____

_____

6. When should you evaluate a client in crisis for suicide risk? (page 192)

_____

_____

_____

_____

_____

7. List nursing diagnoses that often apply to people in crises. (page 195)

_____

_____

_____

_____

_____

8. Have you ever experienced culture shock? List the nursing diagnoses that might have applied to this experience. (pages 192–193)

_____

_____

_____

_____

_____

9. What is the main intent of the crisis intervention model? (pages 195–197)

_____

_____

_____

_____

_____

SELF-ASSESSMENT QUIZ

1. When establishing outcome statements for clients, the nurse would include time frames because (pages 195–196)

    a. they help keep the nurse organized.

    b. time frames can indicate how well a client is managing a crisis.

    c. they identify whether the nurse and client have identified significant problems.

    d. they help to match the appropriate nursing intervention with the client problem.

2. By definition, *crisis* calls for which of the following? (page 182)

    a. Adaptation

    b. Submission

    c. Retreat

    d. Panic

3. The terrorist attacks on September 11, 2001, would be considered which type of crisis? (page 184)

    a. Situational crisis

    b. Maturational crisis

    c. Cultural crisis

    d. Community crisis

4. Studies have found that many survivors of the Buffalo Creek Disaster continue to suffer from (page 188)

    a. depression.

    b. personality disorders.

    c. somatoform disorders.

    d. Post-Traumatic Stress Disorder.

5. Vlahov (2002) found that post-9-11, there was a significant rise in which of the following? (pages 188–189)

    a. Anxiety

    b. Depression

    c. Substance abuse

    d. Personality disorders

6. All of the following are typical responses to stress except (page 185)

    a. adaptation.

    b. fight-flight.

    c. attraction-repulsion.

    d. conservative-withdrawal.

7. Major stressors in today's society include (page 189)

    a. weekends.

    b. television.

    c. drug addiction.

    d. church or temple.

8. The goal of adaptation can be characterized by all the following terms except (pages 190–191)

   a. balance.

   b. equilibrium.

   c. homeostasis.

   d. arousal.

9. All of the following can be effective nursing strategies for a client in crisis except (page 196)

   a. unconditional caring.

   b. allowing for grieving.

   c. pointing out how lucky the client is in other areas of life.

   d. fostering communication about crisis.

10. Which nursing diagnosis would have little application to a client in crisis? (page 195)

   a. Anxiety

   b. Chronic low self-esteem

   c. Dysfunctional grieving

   d. Fear

THE CLIENT EXPERIENCING ANXIETY

The purpose of this chapter is to gain an understanding of when anxiety, which is to some extent a normal part of our everyday lives, becomes problematical and pathological. How can the nurse recognize harmful anxiety, and what nursing care is then appropriate?

READING ASSIGNMENT

Please read Chapter 12, "The Client Experiencing Anxiety," pages 208–250.

KEY TERMS

Write definitions for the following terms in your own words. Compare your definitions with those given in the text.

Adversity_____

_____

Agoraphobia_____

_____

Cognitive-Behavior Therapy_____

_____

Compulsion _____

_____

Fear _____

_____

Generalized Anxiety Disorder_____

_____

Obsession _____

_____

Panic Disorder _____

_____

Phobia_____

_____

Positron Emission Tomography (PET) _____

_____

Post-Traumatic Stress Disorder _____

_____

Trait Anxiety _____

_____

EXERCISES AND ACTIVITIES

1. Review Nursing Tip 12-1 on page 211.

    a. What is the critical difference between fear and anxiety?

    _____

    _____

    _____

    _____

    _____

    b. How is your personal response to fear different from your personal response to anxiety?

    _____

    _____

    _____

    _____

    _____

    c. Can you think of any positive outcomes of fear and anxiety?

_____

_____

_____

_____

_____

2. What are the physiological manifestations of fear and anxiety? Do the two feelings differ in terms of physiological response? (pages 211–212)

_____

_____

_____

_____

_____

3. What do philosophers and writers mean when they characterize the twentieth century as the "age of anxiety"? (page 213)

_____

_____

_____

_____

_____

4. Review Table 12-1, "Stages of Anxiety," on page 214.

    a. What are the differences among the stages?

_____

_____

_____

_____

_____

b. Give an example of each stage.

_____

_____

_____

_____

_____

5. Review Table 12-2, "Summary of Major Anxiety Disorders," on page 215. Test your knowledge by covering one column at a time and verbalizing the hidden information.

6. What are the symptoms of a panic disorder? (pages 216–217)

_____

_____

_____

_____

_____

7. Do you know anyone who experiences a fear of flying? What does this fear have in common with all other phobias? What are the treatment options?

_____

_____

_____

_____

_____

8. Read Nursing Tip 12-3 on page 220. How would you determine if a client in an emergency department were experiencing Social Anxiety Disorder? What kind of therapeutic communication strategies would you employ with such an individual?

_____

_____

_____

_____

_____

9. Review the model for anxiety in Figure 12-1 on page 227.

    a. What is the difference between adversity and trait anxiety?

\
\
\
\
\
\

    b. How would you use this model in your practice?

\
\
\
\
\
\

    c. Do you experience trait anxiety? If not, how do you know? If so, how pronounced is your trait?

\
\
\
\
\
\

10. Table 12-3 on page 229 summarizes data about classes of drugs effective in treating anxiety. List these major classes and note which anxiety disorders are most responsive to each class of drugs.

\
\
\
\
\

11. Many people can point to examples of obsessive or compulsive behavior in their own lives without being diagnosed as having Obsessive-Compulsive Disorder. When do simple repetitive or irresistible behaviors become diagnosable as a disorder? (pages 234–236)

_____

_____

_____

_____

_____

12. Emil F. appears in the emergency department where you work shortly after a gunshot incident in the school where he teaches eighth grade science. Although no one was seriously injured, the incident took place in the classroom next to where Emil was teaching. He is clasping his hands together, and he appears frightened and teary. He states that he has been hyperventilating and cannot seem to regain his composure. He says he is not sure he will be able to return to work.

a. In all likelihood, what is Mr. F. suffering from?

_____

_____

_____

_____

b. What nursing diagnosis would you assess for?

_____

_____

_____

_____

c. What nursing interventions would you perform? What outcomes would be optimal for each intervention?

_____

_____

_____

_____

_____

SELF-ASSESSMENT QUIZ

1. If a client has a fear of an object and is shown a picture of the object, what might be detected when using functional magnetic resonance imaging (fMRI) scanning? (page 212)

   a. Decreased fMRI activity in the amygdala and increased activity in parts of the frontal cortex

   b. Greater fMRI activity in the amygdala and decreased activity in parts of the frontal cortex

   c. Greater fMRI activity in the amygdala and increased activity in parts of the frontal cortex

   d. Decreased fMRI activity in the amygdala and decreased activity in parts of the frontal cortex

2. Many of the peripheral manifestations of fear result in the release of which substance? (page 212)

   a. ACTH

   b. Thyroxin

   c. Gluten

   d. Antidiuretic hormone

3. Many of the evolving treatments for anxiety act as brain receptors for which substance? (page 212)

   a. Dopamine

   b. Serotonin

   c. GABA

   d. ACTH

4. During which stage of anxiety would a person focus on the immediate concern, with a narrowed perceptual field? (page 214)

   a. Mild

   b. Moderate

   c. Severe

   d. Panic

5. Individuals who become acutely anxious when in crowds or when walking through deserted areas are most likely suffering from (pages 217–218)

   a. hydrophobia.

   b. claustrophobia.

   c. agoraphobia.

   d. arachnophobia.

6. The percentage of the population afflicted with phobias is (page 220)

   a. 2%.

   b. 5%.

   c. 10%.

   d. 50%.

7. All of the following are standard treatments for anxiety except (pages 227–230)

   a. psychotherapy.

   b. pharmacotherapy.

   c. behavioral therapy.

   d. isolation therapy.

8. All of the following may contribute to the development of Post-Traumatic Stress Disorder except (pages 224–226)

   a. the degree of the victim's imagination.

   b. the extreme violence of the precipitating event.

   c. poor pre-trauma mental health.

   d. lack of post-trauma support systems.

9. Positron emission tomography (PET) images show the following changes when clients with anxiety disorders are confronted with anxiety-producing stimuli: (page 224)

   a. No changes

   b. Changes in electrical thresholds

   c. Changes in blood flow

   d. Structural changes

Chapter 13

THE CLIENT EXPERIENCING SCHIZOPHRENIA

The purpose of Chapter 13 is to present a vivid clinical picture of the client experiencing schizophrenia. At the same time, the disease is demystified, with a discussion of the range of the illness, its possible causes, its clinical course, treatment, and therapeutic nursing care.

READING ASSIGNMENT

Please read Chapter 13, "The Client Experiencing Schizophrenia," pages 252–286.

KEY TERMS

Write definitions for the following terms in your own words. Compare your definitions with those in the text.

Akathisia _____

_____

Akinesia _____

_____

Alogia _____

_____

Anhedonia _____

_____

Avolition _____

_____

Catatonia_____

_____

Delusion _____

_____

Derailment _____

_____

Dystonia _____

_____

Flattened Affect _____

_____

Grandiose Delusion _____

_____

Hallucination _____

_____

Incoherence _____

_____

Neologistic Word _____

_____

Persecutory Delusion _____

_____

Psychotic _____

_____

Referential Delusion _____

_____

Schizophrenia _____

_____

Tangentiality _____

_____

Tardive Dyskinesia _____

_____

Word Salad _____

_____

EXERCISES AND ACTIVITIES

1. Review the chapter opening on page 252.

   a. Have you thought about what it would be like to care for someone who has a thought disorder?

   _____

   b. How do you plan to prepare yourself for this work?

   _____
   _____
   _____
   _____
   _____

2. Review Box 13-1, "Dispelling Common Myths about Schizophrenia," on page 255.

   a. Did you believe any of these myths? Write a statement that reflects your corrected thinking.

   _____
   _____
   _____
   _____
   _____

   b. Go to the Online Companion for *Psychiatric Mental Health Nursing*, Fourth Edition, located at http://www.delmarlearning.com/companions/ Read the online chapter on dissociative disorders. Did reading this chapter help sharpen your understanding of schizophrenia?

   _____
   _____
   _____
   _____
   _____

3. Read the anonymous "Autobiography" on page 257.

   a. Were you surprised that the author was functioning in a role similar to yours? How much more difficult would your role as a student be if you had schizophrenia?

   _____

   _____

   _____

   _____

   _____

   b. Why do you think this author kept her anonymity?

   _____

   _____

   _____

   _____

   _____

4. Read the three self-reports of delusions on pages 257–258.

   a. Write as many adjectives as come to mind as you read these descriptions. What kind of picture emerges in your mind?

   _____

   _____

   _____

   _____

   _____

   b. How would you respond to a client who reported these delusions to you? What strategies might you use to respond therapeutically?

   _____

   _____

   _____

   _____

   _____

5. Compare and contrast delusions with hallucinations. (pages 257-258)

_____

_____

_____

_____

_____

6. Compare and contrast the positive symptoms of schizophrenia with the negative symptoms of schizophrenia. (pages 258-261)

_____

_____

_____

_____

_____

7. The authors write on page 258 that "some writers and psychiatrists have portrayed persons with schizophrenia as individualistic heroes in a society that celebrates conformity and materialistic values." What is your response to this statement?

_____

_____

_____

_____

_____

8. Examine the PET brain images on page 259. What would you conclude about the brain's ability to differentiate between a hallucination brought about as a result of a psychotic state and the actual experience of the image being hallucinated?

_____

_____

_____

_____

_____

9. Review Figure 13-2, "Genetic Risk for Developing Schizophrenia," on page 264.

    a. What is the risk in the general population of developing schizophrenia?

    _____

    b. According to this figure, what percentage of people with schizophrenia had a parent who had schizophrenia?

    _____

10. State in your own words the current scientific understanding of the cause of schizophrenia. How would you explain to the parent of a teenager recently diagnosed with schizophrenia what the cause is likely to be? (pages 264–266)

    _____

    _____

    _____

    _____

    _____

11. Describe the two major approaches to the treatment of schizophrenia. (pages 239–243)

    _____

    _____

    _____

    _____

    _____

12. Read Nursing Tip 13-1 on page 267.

    a. What nursing needs do families of clients with schizophrenia have?

    _____

    _____

    _____

    _____

    _____

b. What kind of a therapeutic program would you design for families of clients with schizophrenia?

_____

_____

_____

_____

_____

13. Read the discussion of pharmacological treatment of schizophrenia on pages 267–271.

a. Compare and contrast the positives and the negatives associated with treatment of schizophrenia with neuroleptic drugs.

_____

_____

_____

_____

_____

b. Compare second-generation neuroleptics with first-generation neuroleptics.

_____

_____

_____

_____

_____

14. Second-generation neuroleptics are increasingly the drugs of choice for patients with a new diagnosis of schizophrenia.

a. Under what circumstances would a first-generation neuroleptic be a better choice?

_____

_____

_____

_____

    b. What first-generation neuroleptics would be a good choice and under what circumstances?

_____

_____

_____

_____

_____

15. Read the Case Study about "Gary" on page 260. Then, review Table 13-1, "Symptoms Experienced with Schizophrenia and Associated Nursing Diagnoses," on page 271, and the Nursing Diagnosis section on pages 273–280.

    a. Which of these symptoms does Gary seem to suffer?

_____

_____

_____

_____

_____

    b. Write two additional nursing diagnosis statements for Gary, using the information in the Case Study.

_____

_____

_____

_____

_____

16. Classify the following symptoms of schizophrenia according to whether they are positive (P) symptoms or negative (N) symptoms. (pages 256–262)

    a. _____Delusions

    b. _____Lack of motivation

    c. _____Flat affect

d. _____Hallucinations

e. _____Paranoia

f. _____Word salad

g. _____Poor hygiene or grooming

h. _____Poverty of speech

i. _____Poor eye contact

j. _____Grandiose or all-powerful thoughts

k. _____Inability to function

Learning Tip: Positive symptoms are traits "added" to the normal personality, aspects most people don't have, like delusions. Negative symptoms are traits "deleted" from the normal personality, deficits most people don't have, like an inability to function.

17. Compare and contrast the acute and rehabilitative phases of schizophrenia in terms of the following: (page 275)

a. Treatment goals

_____

_____

_____

_____

_____

b. Nurse's role

_____

_____

_____

_____

_____

SELF-ASSESSMENT QUIZ

1. The MRI images of brains from clients with schizophrenia have which of the following differences from brains of clients without schizophrenia? (page 265)

   a. The hippocampus is much larger in clients with schizophrenia.

   b. The ventricles are larger in the clients with schizophrenia.

   c. The hippocampus is much smaller in clients with schizophrenia.

   d. b and c

2. Which two of the following theories have never been seriously considered as the cause of schizophrenia? (pages 263–266)

   a. Genetics

   b. Cause will never be known

   c. Lead poisoning

   d. Inadequate maternal nurturing

   e. Dopamine hypothesis

   f. Phases of the moon

   g. Organic causes

3. Which of the following nursing diagnoses is most likely associated with the rehabilitative phase of schizophrenia? (page 275)

   a. Altered sensory perception

   b. Impaired verbal communication

   c. Ineffective management of therapeutic regimen

   d. Sleep pattern disturbance

4. Which of the following nursing interventions would not be appropriate for managing a client in the rehabilitative phase of schizophrenia? (page 279)

   a. Monitor compliance with medication regime.

   b. Promote social isolation.

   c. Urge client to make a daily schedule and stick with it.

   d. Involve family members in the treatment program.

5. Nurses administering medications on a psychiatric unit know that which of the following are second-generation neuroleptics? (page 270)

    a. Mellaril

    b. Clozapine

    c. Thorazine

    d. Stelazine

6. A client diagnosed with schizophrenia tells the nurse that he does not enjoy the things that used to give him pleasure. The nurse would assess that the client is experiencing which of the following? (pages 258–261)

    a. Anhedonia

    b. Akathesia

    c. Tardive dyskinesia

    d. Dysthymia

7. A nursing instructor evaluates that a nursing student knows the side effects of neuroleptic mediations if the student makes which of the following statements: (pages 268–270)

    a. "Pseudoparkinson symptoms are nonreversible."

    b. "Agranulocytosis can occur when a client receives Thorazine for a long period."

    c. "Tardive dyskinesia is a nonreversible complication of long-term use of first-generation neuroleptics."

    d. "There are very few side effects related to the use of first-generation neuroleptics."

8. The nurse admits a client with a history of schizophrenia. The nursing assessment revealed slowed thinking, flat affect, and lack of motivation. The nurse would interpret this as which of the following? (page 260)

    a. Hallucinations

    b. Delusional behavior

    c. Positive symptoms of schizophrenia

    d. Negative symptoms of schizophrenia

9. Many non-schizophrenic persons display symptoms similar to the negative symptoms of schizophrenia either as part of normal life or as part of another disorder such as (page 260)

   a. anxiety.

   b. depression.

   c. personality disorder.

   d. somatoform disorder.

Chapter 14

THE CLIENT EXPERIENCING DEPRESSION

The purpose of this chapter is to understand the illness of depression in its various forms. Ups, downs, and mood changes are a normal part of life. How dreary and unfulfilling life would be if everyone were cheerful and upbeat all the time! Depressive disorders occur when the downswings in mood are deep, unrelenting, and dysfunctional. Learning to recognize and respond to depression is an essential skill for nurses because depression is a pervasive and devastating illness frequently seen in clients hospitalized for other medical reasons.

READING ASSIGNMENT

Please read Chapter 14, "The Client Experiencing Depression," pages 288–331.

KEY TERMS

Write definitions for the following terms in your own words. Compare your definitions with those given in the text.

Bipolar Depression _____

_____

Chronic Grief _____

_____

Cognitive Therapy _____

_____

Delayed Grief _____

_____

Depression _____

_____

Ego _____

_____

Emotion-Focused Therapy _____

_____

Exaggerated Grief _____

_____

Grief _____

_____

Marital Therapy _____

_____

Masked Grief _____

_____

Mood Disorder _____

_____

Mood Episode _____

_____

Nurse Agency _____

_____

Self-Care Agency _____

_____

Superego _____

_____

Supportive-Educative Role _____

_____

Unipolar Depression _____

_____

EXERCISES AND ACTIVITIES

1. Much of the important content of this chapter has to do with diagnosing depression and differentiating it from the normal ups and downs of daily experience. (pages 292–299)

   a. Describe the difference between a Minor Depressive Disorder and a Major Depressive Disorder.

   _____

   _____

   _____

   _____

   _____

   b. Describe the difference between a Major Depressive Episode and a Major Depressive Disorder.

   _____

   _____

   _____

   _____

   _____

   c. What are the major symptoms of depression?

   _____

   _____

   _____

   _____

   _____

d. What factors and symptoms must be present for there to be a diagnosis of Major Depressive Disorder?

_____

_____

_____

_____

_____

e. Describe the differences between Major Depressive Disorder and Dysthymic Disorder.

_____

_____

_____

_____

_____

f. Describe the differences between depression and grief.

_____

_____

_____

_____

_____

2. Read the material about Post-Partum Depression. (pages 296–297)

a. What risk factors seem to be associated with Post-Partum Depression?

_____

_____

_____

_____

_____

b. What factors do *not* seem to be risk factors for Post-Partum Depression?

_____

_____

_____

_____

_____

c. What nursing interventions may be effective in assessing and treating Post-Partum Depression?

_____

_____

_____

_____

_____

3. List the risk factors for depression. (page 297)

_____

_____

_____

_____

_____

4. List the theories of depression. (pages 299–302)

_____

_____

_____

_____

_____

   a. To which theory do you most subscribe, and why?

_____

_____

_____

_____

_____

   b. Which other theories merit serious evaluation, in your view, and why?

_____

_____

_____

_____

_____

5. Describe the stages of bereavement. (pages 297–299)

_____

_____

_____

_____

_____

6. Have you experienced the death of a loved one in your life?

   a. Describe your grief response, relating it to the stages you identified previously.

_____

_____

_____

_____

_____

    b. How would you evaluate successful grieving in yourself or in a client you are treating?

_____

_____

_____

_____

_____

7. Identify the four types of dysfunctional grieving, and describe their unique characteristics. (page 299)

_____

_____

_____

_____

_____

8. Identify the two lasting contributions of psychoanalysis to our current understanding of depression. (pages 299–300)

_____

_____

_____

_____

_____

9. What is *Bowlby's controversy*, and what is your view of the issue? (page 300)

_____

_____

_____

_____

_____

10. What are the three types of treatment for depression? (pages 302–308)

_____

_____

_____

_____

_____

   a. Compare and contrast the effectiveness of these three treatment types.

   _____

   _____

   _____

   _____

   _____

   b. What kinds of clients make the best candidates for each of the three types of treatment?

   _____

   _____

   _____

   _____

   _____

11. Name the three classes of medication generally used to treat depression. (pages 304–308)

_____

_____

_____

a. Identify the strengths of each class of medication.

_____

_____

_____

_____

_____

b. Identify the drawbacks of each class of medication.

_____

_____

_____

_____

_____

c. What education would you provide for clients taking each class of medication?

_____

_____

_____

_____

_____

12. Identify the nursing diagnoses commonly used for clients with depression. (page 312) Be sure to differentiate between the two diagnoses related to grieving.

_____

_____

_____

_____

_____

13. What advice would you give clients who want to use St. John's wort (*Hypericum*) to treat their depression?

_____

_____

_____

_____

_____

SELF-ASSESSMENT QUIZ

1. Which of the following is an over-the-counter drug used to treat depression? (page 308)

    a. Gingko biloba

    b. Black kohash

    c. St. John's wort

    d. Linseed oil

2. A priority assessment for clients with major depression would be which of the following? (page 308)

    a. Risk for depression

    b. Altered nutritional status

    c. Ability to form strong interpersonal relationships

    d. Response to currently prescribed medications

3. Normal sunlight would be most effective in treating which of the following disorders? (page 304)

    a. Dysthymia

    b. Bipolar Disorder

    c. Seasonal Affective Disorder

    d. Psychotic Depression

4. For a Major Depressive Episode to count toward the diagnosis of Major Depressive Disorder, it must have all the following characteristics except (page 282)

    a. it must cause the client to be sleepy and irritable.

    b. it must last at least two weeks.

    c. it must represent a change from previous functioning.

    d. it must interfere with the client's ability to function in a social or occupational situation.

5. Risk factors associated with depression include all the following except (page 297)

    a. recent negative life stressors.

    b. confusion.

    c. significant physical disease.

    d. family history of depression.

6. For cases of treatment-resistant depression, the treatment proven most effective is (page 303)

    a. allowing time to pass.

    b. electroconvulsive therapy (ECT).

    c. Prozac.

    d. MAO inhibitors.

7. All of the following classes of medications are used to treat depression except (pages 304–308)

    a. tricyclics.

    b. amphetamines.

    c. MAO inhibitors.

    d. selective serotonin reuptake inhibitors.

8. Clinical problems associated with the use of tricyclics include all of the following except (pages 305–306)

    a. they are often fatal in an overdose, making them problematic for clients who may be suicidal.

    b. orthostatic side effects.

    c. they frequently cause insomnia and other sleep disturbances.

    d. anticholinergic side effects.

9. Some recent findings of nursing research include all of the following except (page 313)

    a. exercise can be an effective antidepressant.

    b. cognitive therapy can have an antidepressant effect.

    c. the ability to perform self-care has a positive effect on mood.

    d. depressed women from low socioeconomic backgrounds have a better prognosis than depressed women of affluent means.

10. All of the following nursing interventions are helpful to clients with depression except (page 314)

    a. providing overhead light 24 hours per day.

    b. cultural assessments.

    c. movement therapy.

    d. understanding the client's subjective experience of depression and pain.

11. Which of the following statements about St. John's wort (*Hypericum*) is not true? (page 308)

    a. Some patients may be more open to taking it than standard antidepressants.

    b. St. John's wort has been shown to be as effective as drug therapy or cognitive therapy.

    c. St. John's wort may help trigger mania in patients with unrecognized Manic-Depressive Disease.

    d. St. John's wort is an extract of a natural botanical.

12. **Identify the following drugs as tricyclics (T), SSRIs (S), or MAOIs (M). (pages 304–308)**

    a. _____ Elavil

    b. _____ Sinequan

    c. _____ Parnate

    d. _____ Prozac

    e. _____ Anafranil

    f. _____ Nardil

    g. _____ Paxil

    h. _____ Pamelor

    i. _____ Zoloft

    j. _____ Tofranil

Chapter 15

THE CLIENT EXPERIENCING MANIA

The purpose of this chapter is to gain an understanding of mania in all its forms, cycles, and manifestations. Just as depression should not be confused with the lows that sometimes accompany daily life, neither should mania be confused with the happiness, elation, and cheerfulness that all of us normally experience. When is mania pathological, and what is the nursing care associated with this complex mental illness?

READING ASSIGNMENT

Please read Chapter 15, "The Client Experiencing Mania," pages 332–367

KEY TERMS

Write definitions for the following terms in your own words. Compare your definitions with those given in the text.

Bipolar Disorder (BPD) _____

_____

Borderline Personality _____

_____

Continuous Cycling _____

_____

Cyclothymic Pattern _____

_____

Grandiosity _____

_____

Hypomania _____

_____

Mania _____

_____

Manic Episode _____

_____

Rapid Cycling_____

_____

Schizoaffective Disorder_____

_____

Switch Process_____

_____

EXERCISES AND ACTIVITIES

1. In one minute, list as many adjectives as you can to describe mania.

    _____

    _____

    _____

    _____

    _____

2. Study Table 15-1, "Stages of Mania," on page 335.

    a. Cover the columns under Stage I, Stage II, and Stage III to make sure you know how mood, cognition, and behavior change as the client moves among the stages.

    b. Identify a television character you have seen with each of the three stages of mania.

    _____

    _____

    _____

c. The authors state that studies on the efficacy of treatment should focus more on the client's perception of benefit, not on whether the DSM-IV-TR-based diagnostic criteria have been met. Do you agree or disagree? Why?

_____

_____

_____

_____

_____

3. List the manic behaviors necessary for a diagnosis of a manic episode. (page 336)

_____

_____

_____

_____

_____

4. Differentiate among the three diagnoses of manic episode, hypomania, and Bipolar Disorder. (pages 336–337)

_____

_____

_____

_____

_____

5. Review Figure 15-1, "Clinical Course of Mania," on page 338.

a. What conclusions can you draw about the frequency of episodes?

_____

_____

_____

_____

_____

b. What conclusions can you draw about the frequency, timing, and effect of hospitalizations?

_____

_____

_____

_____

_____

6. Review Figure 15-2, "Psychologic Genealogy: Family with Bipolar and Depressive Disease," on page 340.

a. What conclusions can you draw about the nature and cause of bipolar disease?

_____

_____

_____

_____

_____

b. According to the genealogy, in the original marriage between Elizabeth (Clayton) and Michael (Tennyson) that united the two families, the couple themselves lived free of mental illness. What significance has this had on their descendents?

_____

_____

_____

_____

_____

c. What other evidence suggests that bipolar disease is genetic and biologically based?

_____

_____

_____

_____

_____

7. What other factors can cause manic-like symptoms? (pages 342–343)

_____

_____

_____

_____

_____

8. Complicating the diagnosis of mania is the possibility of dual diagnosis. What psychiatric conditions seem to travel in tandem with mania, making the diagnosis more problematical? (pages 343–344)

_____

_____

_____

_____

_____

9. Describe the pharmacological treatment of mania. (pages 344–349)

_____

_____

_____

_____

_____

a. List the benefits of lithium.

_____

_____

_____

_____

_____

b. List the drawbacks of lithium.

_____

_____

_____

_____

_____

c. Explain the role of antipsychotics, particularly the newer atypical or second-generation antipsychotics, in the treatment of bipolar illness.

_____

_____

_____

_____

_____

d. Explain the role of antidepressants in the treatment of bipolar illness.

_____

_____

_____

_____

10. If you were in charge of an inpatient setting and wanted to create a therapeutic milieu for clients with Bipolar Disorder, what features would you establish? (page 351) Think about limits, space, schedules, privileges, medication regimens, and other elements of a therapeutic milieu.

_____

_____

_____

_____

_____

SELF-ASSESSMENT QUIZ

1. One of the most interesting ideas to emerge from genetic studies is a possible linkage between which of the following disorders? (page 341)

    a. Bipolar psychosis and chemical abuse

    b. Bipolar psychosis and schizophrenia

    c. Bipolar psychosis and somatoform disorders

    d. Bipolar psychosis and personality disorders

2. Use of which of the following as an adjunct to smoking cessation is much less likely to cause manic switch? (page 343)

    a. Brupropion

    b. BuSpar

    c. Benzodiazepine

    d. Betadine

3. Which of the following has a higher potential for toxicity? (pages 344–345)

    a. Lithium

    b. Olanzapine

    c. Valprorate

    d. Clozapine

4. Which of the following antipsychotics has the lowest potential of being associated with weight gain? (page 348)

    a. Haldol

    b. Thorazine

    c. Clozapine

    d. Ziprasidone

5. A recent study has shown that those with bipolar disorder lose approximately how many workdays per year as a result of severe depression? (page 342)

   a. 15

   b. 35

   c. 65

   d. 95

6. The clinical course for people with bipolar disease can vary among all the following except (page 342)

   a. rapid cycling.

   b. mania with no depression.

   c. continuous cycling.

   d. mostly depression.

7. Dual diagnoses often associated with mania include all of the following except (pages 343–344)

   a. Sociopathic Personality Disorder.

   b. substance abuse.

   c. Borderline Personality Disorder.

   d. Schizoaffective Disorder.

8. The primary treatment for Bipolar Disorder is (page 344)

   a. psychotherapy.

   b. hospitalization and milieu therapy.

   c. channeling.

   d. medication.

9. Nursing interventions appropriate for clients with mania might include all of the following except (page 353)

   a. milieu therapy.

   b. insight-oriented counseling and teaching about the disease when clients are between manic episodes.

   c. insight-oriented counseling and teaching about the disease when clients are experiencing manic episodes.

   d. encouraging clients to consider the benefits of lithium therapy.

10. Parse's Theory of Human Becoming views disease as a normal part of life, something that has to be interpreted by the client, who must find individual meaning in disease as well as in health. For a nurse who approaches clinical work from this theoretical viewpoint, all of the following would be appropriate interventions except which approach? (page 350)

    a. Make no demands on the client.

    b. Help the client find and prioritize personal values.

    c. Help the client accept the health team's treatment plan.

    d. Try to understand the client's world and use that understanding to gain trust and collaboration.

11. All of the following are signs of mania except (page 334)

    a. increased sexual activity.

    b. spending sprees.

    c. carefully planned suicide attempts.

    d. grandiose thinking.

12. The nursing assessment of a client diagnosed with hypomania would most likely reveal which of the following? (page 336)

    a. Pressured speech, talkativeness, and flight of ideas

    b. Lack of motivation, delusional thinking, and low self-esteem

    c. Positive self-concept, decreased motivation, and depression

    d. Anhedonia, blunted affect, and waxy flexibility

13. Which of the following nursing interventions would take priority for a client in a manic state? (page 353)

    a. Placing the client in restraints

    b. Setting limits on the client's behavior

    c. Having the client play a competitive game with another client

    d. Encouraging the client to read a novel

Chapter 16

THE CLIENT WHO IS SUICIDAL

The purpose of this chapter is to learn to identify clients who are at risk of suicide. Even clients who experience suicidal ideation or who make suicidal gestures to gain attention can unintentionally kill themselves in a momentary impulse or miscalculation. While suicide is associated with some disorders more than others, a wide variety of mental and physical illnesses can make people feel so awful that they might consider suicide.

READING ASSIGNMENT

Please read Chapter 16, "The Client Who Is Suicidal," pages 368–402.

KEY TERMS

Write definitions for the following terms in your own words. Compare your definitions with those given in the text.

Euthanasia _____

_____

Suicidal Ideation _____

_____

Suicide _____

_____

Suicide Potential _____

_____

Suicide Survivor _____

_____

EXERCISES AND ACTIVITIES

1. Who is at risk for suicide? Identify as many groups at risk discussed in this chapter as you can.

_____

_____

_____

_____

_____

2. There are conflicting data over what percentage of people who commit suicide have a major mental illness. (page 371) After reading the chapter, what is your view?

_____

_____

_____

_____

_____

3. Nurses must be able to assess a client's potential to commit suicide. What risk factors and other conditions and circumstances can you list as concerns to assess for? (page 372)

_____

_____

_____

_____

4. Peplau's Theory of Interpersonal Relations in nursing stresses the importance of forming therapeutic relationships with clients. How can you use this nursing knowledge to reduce the likelihood of clients attempting suicide? (pages 377–378)

_____

_____

_____

_____

_____

5. What precautions can the nurse take to protect hospitalized clients from hurting themselves? (pages 390–391)

_____

_____

_____

_____

_____

6. What precautions can the nurse take to protect clients in the community from hurting themselves? (pages 372–375)

_____

_____

_____

_____

_____

7. Describe the three levels of prevention for suicide. (pages 387–389)

_____

_____

_____

_____

_____

8. In comparing prisoners and members of the military to the general U.S. population, what conclusions can you draw about these groups' suicide risk?

_____

_____

_____

_____

_____

9. After reading this chapter, has your attitude changed toward the following issues? If so, in what ways? (pages 389–391)

   a. Gun control

_____

_____

_____

_____

_____

   b. Assisted suicide

_____

_____

_____

_____

_____

   c. Accident rates (which may inadvertently include intentional self-harm)

_____

_____

_____

_____

_____

10. Study Vincent Van Gogh's last painting on page 379.

    a. Do you agree with the authors' view of elements in the painting that signify death?

    _____

    _____

    _____

    _____

    _____

    b. Would you be concerned if a depressed client showed you a recent painting with some of the features the author identified in Van Gogh's *Wheatfield with Crows*?

    _____

    _____

    _____

    _____

    _____

    c. In what other ways do suicidal clients frequently convey their morbid thoughts of death?

    _____

    _____

    _____

    _____

    _____

SELF-ASSESSMENT QUIZ

1. Which of the following individuals is most at risk for suicide? (page 371)

    a. A male 15–19 years old

    b. A female 35–40 years old

    c. A female 56–60 years old

    d. A male 75–80 years old

2. Completed suicide rates have dropped significantly in a number of countries over the past decade, especially for which group? (page 371)

    a. Infants

    b. Children and adolescents

    c. Young adults

    d. Older adults

3. According to World Health Organization (WHO) data, what percentage of individuals worldwide who commit suicide had a psychiatric diagnosis at the time of death? (page 372)

    a. 25%

    b. 48%

    c. 73%

    d. 90%

4. In 2007, politically and religiously motivated murders-suicides accounted for how many deaths in Afghanistan? (page 374)

    a. 500

    b. 1,100

    c. 1,700

    d. 2,500

5. A study on the characteristics of patients being treated for attempted suicide in hospital emergency departments revealed that the most commonly used method of self-harm was which of the following? (page 376)

    a. Cuts and other stab wounds

    b. Drug/medication overdose

    c. Attempted suffocation or drowning

    d. Use of a small-caliber pistol

6. Explanations of suicide include all of the following except (pages 375–378)

   a. Kevorkian theory.

   b. sociological theory.

   c. psychological theory.

   d. biological theory.

7. The major psychiatric diagnosis most frequently associated with suicide is (pages 372–375)

   a. Major Depressive Disorder.

   b. schizophrenia.

   c. Antisocial Personality Disorder.

   d. hypochondriasis.

8. Primary prevention of suicide includes all of the following interventions except (pages 388–390)

   a. being aware of which groups are at greatest risk of committing suicide.

   b. limiting access to the means of suicide.

   c. using crisis intervention techniques.

   d. reducing the client's social isolation.

9. A "suicide contract" is (page 391)

   a. a signed agreement between a nurse and a client in which the client promises not to commit suicide during a specific period of time.

   b. a suicide pact.

   c. a client's verbal agreement to never commit suicide without first notifying the nurse.

   d. an exclusion in a life insurance policy.

10. Tobacco use is associated with increased risk of suicide in (page 375)

   a. both men and women.

   b. just men.

   c. just women.

   d. none of the above.

Chapter 17

THE CLIENT WHO ABUSES CHEMICAL SUBSTANCES

The purpose of this chapter is to present the psychiatric implications of substance abuse. By concentrating on the four most pervasively abused substances, though there are others, nurses can familiarize themselves with the dynamics of abuse and addiction, the effects on clients and their families, and the nursing care associated with clients who abuse substances.

READING ASSIGNMENT

Please read Chapter 17, "The Client Who Abuses Chemical Substances," pages 404-449.

KEY TERMS

Write definitions for the following terms in your own words. Compare definitions with those given in the text.

Addiction _____

_____

Alcoholism _____

_____

Codependence_____

_____

Craving _____

_____

Drug Dependence _____

_____

Drug Use_____

_____

Substance Abuse _____

_____

Tolerance _____

_____

Withdrawal_____

_____

EXERCISES AND ACTIVITIES

1. Terminology associated with drug abuse can be imprecise and confusing. (page 407)

    a. Explain why the DSM-IV-TR uses the phrase *physiological dependence* rather than *addiction*.

        _____

        _____

        _____

        _____

        _____

    b. Explain the concept of tolerance.

        _____

        _____

        _____

        _____

        _____

    c. Explain the concept of withdrawal.

        _____

        _____

        _____

        _____

        _____

2. The text details efforts made by governments over the centuries to control the supply of drugs. (pages 409–410)

   a. In your view, which, if any, of these measures has proven effective?

   _____

   _____

   _____

   _____

   _____

   b. Besides limiting supply, governments can also act to limit demand. What efforts have governments made to limit demand?

   _____

   _____

   _____

   _____

   _____

   c. Have any such efforts been successful?

   _____

   _____

   _____

   _____

   _____

3. In recent years, as virtually all hospitals have become "no-smoking" zones, nurses have had to manage the problem of nicotine-dependent psychiatric clients who, already stressed by their primary diseases, must also abstain from smoking. (pages 410–411)

    a. What specific stressors does this add to the client's burden?

_____

_____

_____

_____

_____

    b. As a nurse, what can you do to help the client through this transition?

_____

_____

_____

_____

_____

4. What are the long-term adverse physical effects of chronic alcohol abuse? (pages 412–415)

_____

_____

_____

_____

_____

5. The first task of treating clients with alcoholism is to help them withdraw from their physiological dependence on alcohol. (pages 415–419)

    a. Describe the typical human response to alcohol withdrawal.

_____

_____

_____

_____

_____

b. Describe the usual medical regimen for managing the client during alcohol withdrawal.

_____

_____

_____

_____

_____

c. Describe measures nurses can take to help the client cope with alcohol withdrawal and the period immediately following withdrawal.

_____

_____

_____

_____

_____

6. Describe the natural history of alcoholism. (page 416)

_____

_____

_____

_____

_____

7. Disulfiram (Antabuse) continues to be used in treating alcoholism. (page 417)

a. Describe its mechanism.

_____

_____

_____

_____

_____

b. What have been the drawbacks of disulfiram?

_____

_____

_____

_____

_____

c. What other drugs are frequently used to treat people with alcoholism, and what are their indications?

_____

_____

_____

_____

_____

8. Describe the nursing "Brief Intervention" using the FRAMES Model. (page 419)

_____

_____

_____

_____

_____

9. Over the years, the medical community has taken a somewhat "permissive" stance toward the use of cocaine. (pages 419–421)

a. What are the true medical consequences of regular cocaine use?

_____

_____

_____

_____

_____

b. What is the DSM-IV-TR's stance on the danger of cocaine? (page 422)

_____

_____

_____

_____

_____

10. Review the treatment options for clients with opiate dependence. (pages 424–426)

   a. What is the central decision clinicians must make in choosing a treatment for a person addicted to opiates?

   _____

   _____

   _____

   _____

   _____

   b. Summarize the pros and cons of methadone maintenance therapy.

   _____

   _____

   _____

   _____

   _____

   c. What is your personal opinion of methadone maintenance therapy?

   _____

   _____

   _____

   _____

   _____

11. Many public policy options are available in response to the social problem of substance abuse, ranging from long prison terms (and, in some countries, even executions) for drug users to total legalization of all chemical substances. (page 428) In your own words, state the policy you think our country should pursue.

_____

_____

_____

_____

_____

SELF-ASSESSMENT QUIZ

1. A client is detoxing from cocaine abuse. The nurse would assess for which of the following major complications of cocaine withdrawal? (page 420)

   a. Renal failure

   b. Constipation

   c. Cardiac arrhythmias

   d. Muscle weakness

2. The nurse would assess for which of the following in a client who has experienced cannabis intoxication? (page 427)

   a. Drowsiness and anorexia

   b. Euphoria, dry mouth, and sensation of slowing time

   c. Bradycardia, drowsiness, and difficulty breathing

   d. Euphoria, anorexia, and vomiting

3. Which of the following medications stimulates and blocks nicotine-binding receptors and is effective in treating clients who want to quit smoking? (page 411)

   a. Varenicline

   b. Thorazine

   c. Apresoline

   d. Cimetidine

4. Studies have found that what percentage of RNs and LPNs smoke? (pages 411–412)

    a. 1% of RNs and 10% of LPNs

    b. 6% of RNs and 18% of LPNs

    c. 15% of RNs and 28% of LPNs

    d. 25% of RNs and 9% of LPNs

5. Which of the following anticonvulsants appears to have some benefit in reducing craving and promoting abstinence from cocaine? (page 422)

    a. Phenobarbital

    b. Dilantin

    c. Carbamazepine

    d. Topiramate

6. Among the following substances, which is not identified in the DSM-IV-TR as a dependency psychiatric condition? (page 408)

    a. Cannabis

    b. Alcohol

    c. Caffeine

    d. Nicotine

7. *Codependence* refers to the relationship between (page 431)

    a. the addict and his or her dealer.

    b. two addicts or abusers.

    c. an abuser and the significant other who facilitates the substance abuse.

    d. the nurse and the substance abuser.

8. All of the following are classified as stimulants except (page 408)

    a. nicotine.

    b. cocaine.

    c. alcohol.

    d. caffeine.

9. New tests identifying persons at risk for alcohol abuse (Carbohydrate Deficient Transferrin, Early Detection of Alcohol Consumption tests) are rarely used because (page 415)

    a. they're not approved by the FDA.

    b. nurses and other clinicians often don't know about them.

    c. they're too costly.

    d. they have unpleasant side effects.

    e. a and d

    f. b and c

    g. b and d

10. A recovering alcoholic should be counseled to do all of the following except (page 416)

    a. attend AA meetings.

    b. learn how to say no to drinking alcohol at a party.

    c. deal with problems caused by drinking over the years.

    d. spend time in drinking establishments to test one's ability not to drink anymore.

Chapter 18

THE CLIENT WITH A PERSONALITY DISORDER

The purpose of this chapter is to better understand the concept of personality by first examining normal personality and then defects in personalities. You will learn about eleven personality disorders clustered within three types and how to be effective in providing nursing care to individuals with a personality disorder.

READING ASSIGNMENT

Please read Chapter 18, "The Client with a Personality Disorder," pages 450-493.

KEY TERMS

Write definitions for the following terms in your own words. Compare your definitions with those given in the text.

Antisocial Personality Disorder _____

_____

Avoidant Personality Disorder _____

_____

Borderline Personality Disorder _____

_____

Dependent Personality Disorder _____

_____

Histrionic Personality Disorder _____

_____

Narcissistic Personality Disorder _____

_____

Obsessive-Compulsive Personality Disorder _____

_____

Paranoid Personality Disorder_____

_____

Passive-Aggressive Personality Disorder_____

_____

Personality _____

_____

Personality Disorder _____

_____

Personality Traits _____

_____

Schizoid Personality Disorder_____

_____

Schizotypal Personality Disorder _____

_____

EXERCISES AND ACTIVITIES

1. Personality disorders are considered Axis II disorders in the DSM-IV-TR, whereas most major mental illnesses are Axis I disorders. Explain the relationship between Axis II and Axis I disorders and the significance of these classifications. (page 452)

   _____

   _____

   _____

   _____

   _____

2. Almost all of us have some personality traits associated with a personality disorder. What is necessary for an individual to be diagnosed with a personality disorder? (page 453)

_____

_____

_____

_____

_____

3. Review Table 18-1, "Personality Disorders by Descriptive Category," on page 453.

   a. What are the three clusters of personality disorders?

   _____

   _____

   _____

   _____

   _____

   b. How are these clusters categorized?

   _____

   _____

   _____

   _____

4. Early psychiatrists coined the term *borderline personality* because of their observations that these usually "neurotic" individuals often lived their lives on the "borderline" between neurosis and psychosis, particularly when experiencing stress. Under stress, these individuals frequently plunge into delusions, hallucinations, paranoia, and fantasies that, although they may not be persistent, are definitely psychotic. (page 456)

a. List the characteristics necessary for an individual to be diagnosed with Borderline Personality Disorder.

_____

_____

_____

_____

_____

b. Identify the typical characteristics of the childhood and home life of a person diagnosed with Borderline Personality Disorder.

_____

_____

_____

_____

_____

c. Clients with Borderline Personality Disorder can be challenging to care for. They tend to focus anger on their caregivers and blame others for their problems. They often try to "split" staff and tend to regard nurses as either allies or enemies. Since part of their illness involves a failure to form healthy relationships in their lives, it may not be surprising that they can be hard to like, and it can be hard to develop trusting therapeutic relationships with them. Considering all this, what strategies would you use to provide therapeutic nursing care to such a person?

_____

_____

_____

_____

_____

5. Consider the personality disorders of the dramatic and emotional cluster. (pages 453–463)

    a. What is the key difference between Borderline Personality Disorder and Narcissistic Personality Disorder?

    _____

    _____

    _____

    _____

    _____

    b. What are the similarities between Borderline Personality Disorder and Histrionic Personality Disorder?

    _____

    _____

    _____

    _____

    _____

    c. What is the key difference between Borderline Personality Disorder and Histrionic Personality Disorder?

    _____

    _____

    _____

    _____

    _____

d. People with Narcissistic Personality Disorder and people with Histrionic Personality Disorder grow up with an exaggerated sense of the importance of good looks. What life events do you think would tend to precipitate crises in these individuals? Would you expect people with the two disorders to respond any differently to these stressors?

_____

_____

_____

_____

_____

e. Clients with any of the dramatic and emotional personality disorders can place great demands on the nurse and try to use the nurse as an object in their effort to get their dysfunctional needs met. As a nurse, what strategies can you employ to minimize the demanding quality of people with these disorders?

_____

_____

_____

_____

_____

f. Although it is imperative not to stereotype individuals just because they have been diagnosed according to a set group of traits or behaviors, there is empirical evidence to show that people with Borderline Personality Disorder are more often women and people with Antisocial Personality Disorder are more often men. Do you think this trend will change as gender roles continue to evolve in society at large?

_____

_____

_____

_____

_____

6. Review the text material on the odd and eccentric cluster of personality disorders. (pages 463-469)

a. What are the essential differences between Schizoid Personality Disorder and schizophrenia?

_____

_____

_____

_____

_____

b. What is the essential difference between Schizotypal Personality Disorder and schizophrenia?

_____

_____

_____

_____

_____

c. In your own words, explain the difference between Schizoid Personality Disorder and Schizoptypal Personality Disorder.

_____

_____

_____

_____

_____

7. Characterize the difference between paranoid schizophrenia and Paranoid Personality Disorder. (page 467)

_____

_____

_____

_____

_____

8. Characterize the difference between Obsessive-Compulsive Personality Disorder and Obsessive-Compulsive Disorder, an anxiety disorder. (page 470)

_____

_____

_____

_____

_____

9. The difference between being shy and being diagnosed with Avoidant Personality Disorder is a question of degree. How would you identify the personality disorder as opposed to the personality trait? (pages 471–474)

_____

_____

_____

_____

_____

10. Have you known people who have a "passive-aggressive" style? (pages 476–477) Almost everyone has. What kinds of strategies have you developed to deal with such people?

_____

_____

_____

_____

_____

11. Read Research Highlight 18-1, "To Tame a Volcano," on page 457.

   a. If you were to develop a study related to the suffering of clients with Borderline Personality Disorder, how would your research design differ?

   _____

   _____

   _____

   _____

   _____

   b. Would your subjects be different in terms of age and gender? If so, explain why.

   _____

   _____

   _____

   _____

SELF-ASSESSMENT QUIZ

1. Personality disorders generally develop during (page 452)

   a. infancy.

   b. childhood.

   c. adolescence.

   d. late adulthood.

2. The most common of the odd cluster personality disorders is (page 466)

   a. Paranoid Personality Disorder.

   b. Schizotypal Personality Disorder.

   c. Narcissistic Personality Disorder.

   d. Schizoid Personality Disorder.

3. Which of the following personality disorders was removed from the DSM-IV, but later included in the DSM-IV-TR as a category requiring further study? (page 453)

   a. Dependent Personality Disorder

   b. Antisocial Personality Disorder

   c. Obsessive-Compulsive Personality Disorder

   d. Passive-Aggressive Personality Disorder

4. Which of the following statements is true regarding personality disorders? (page 452)

   a. Personality disorders are illnesses or conditions that a person acquires at some point in his or her life.

   b. Personality disorders are illnesses that develop during adulthood.

   c. Personality disorders are descriptions of the characteristics that an individual has and expresses that make up the whole of who the individual is.

   d. Personality disorders are conditions that are most effectively treated with intense psychoanalysis and antipsychotic medications.

5. Dialectic behavior therapy usually involves (page 456)

   a. once-weekly individual therapy sessions and twice-weekly group sessions, along with crisis interventions.

   b. twice-weekly individual therapy sessions and once-weekly group sessions, along with antidepressant medications.

   c. three weekly individual therapy sessions, including antipsychotic medications.

   d. three group therapy sessions, one family therapy session weekly, combined with antidepressant medication.

6. For an individual to be diagnosed with a personality disorder, all of the following must be present except (pages 452–476)

   a. the individual must experience clinically significant distress or impairment.

   b. the cluster of traits must be consistent with the diagnosis.

   c. the personality disorder cluster of traits must be pervasive and inflexible.

   d. personality traits must often lead to hostility and conflict.

7. Strategies a nurse might use to deal with the demanding quality of clients with dramatic and emotional personality disorders include all of the following except (pages 476–477)

    a. setting limits on the time you devote to these clients' demands.

    b. communicating with colleagues to ensure a consistent approach toward these clients.

    c. giving these clients a little extra attention so there will be a positive feeling between you and them.

    d. responding to these clients' needs in a professional, efficient manner.

8. An effective nursing response to clients with Schizoid Personality Disorder and Schizoptypal Personality Disorder might include any of the following except (page 465)

    a. designing a behavior modification program to improve social skills and increase inventory of expressive traits.

    b. accepting clients for themselves.

    c. giving clients honest feedback on how their behavior is seen by others.

    d. relating to clients in a professional, matter-of-fact manner, knowing that developing a normal relationship is inconsistent with the nature of their illness.

9. In caring for a person with a Paranoid Personality Disorder, the nurse should not attempt to (page 469)

    a. respond to the client in an unemotional way.

    b. focus on the major features of the client's dysfunctional behavior.

    c. try to convince the client that paranoid feelings are unfounded.

    d. give honest feedback to the client on how the client's behavior is perceived by others.

10. When caring for a person with a personality disorder, nurses should keep in mind all of the following except which? (pages 479–481)

    a. Clients with personality disorders may not be as likable as other clients with fully integrated personalities, requiring nurses to compensate for their personality deficits.

    b. Clients with personality disorders respond best to clear expectations as expressed in contracts, schedules, responsibilities, and limits.

    c. Clients with personality disorders benefit from honest feedback.

    d. Clients with personality disorders benefit from having faithful allies on the nursing staff.

Chapter 19

THE CLIENT EXPERIENCING A SOMATOFORM, FACTITIOUS, OR DISSOCIATIVE DISORDER

The purpose of this chapter is to understand a complex group of disorders that have the symptoms of physical diseases but have causes that lie in the psychological realm. These clients present special challenges to nursing care. They often demand that a diagnosis be made when in fact there is none to be made, and then they view their caretakers as incompetent for not curing the physical "disease." They are often unable to gain insight into their true conditions; yet, they actually feel ill—and ill treated.

READING ASSIGNMENT

Please read Chapter 19, "The Client Experiencing a Somatoform, Factitious, or Dissociative Disorder," pages 494–524.

KEY TERMS

Write definitions for the following terms in your own words. Compare your definitions with those given in the text.

Amnesia _____

_____

Conversion Disorder _____

_____

Depersonalization _____

_____

Dissociative Disorders _____

_____

Dissociative Identity Disorder (DID) _____

_____

Factitious Disorder _____

_____

Fugue _____

_____

Hypochondriasis _____

_____

Malingering _____

_____

Munchausen's Syndrome _____

_____

Munchausen's Syndrome by Proxy _____

_____

Somatization Disorder _____

_____

Somatoform Disorder _____

_____

EXERCISES AND ACTIVITIES

1. Name the four classes of disorders discussed in this chapter, briefly distinguishing one from another.

_____

_____

_____

_____

_____

2. Somatoform disorder was once called "hysteria." (pages 497–498)

   a. What is the difference between somatoform disorder and hysteria?

   _____

   _____

   _____

   _____

   _____

   b. Why is the term *hysteria* not used in the language of psychology anymore?

   _____

   _____

   _____

   _____

   _____

3. List the four criteria for diagnosing someone with Somatization Disorder. (page 498)

   _____

   _____

   _____

   _____

   _____

4. Treatment of Somatization Disorder is notoriously difficult and frequently ineffective. Describe the nursing care that is usually associated with and sometimes effective for this disorder. (page 501)

   _____

   _____

   _____

   _____

   _____

5. What are the diagnostic criteria for hypochondriasis? (pages 502–503)

_____

_____

_____

_____

_____

   a. How is hypochondriasis different from the anxiety disorders?

     _____

     _____

     _____

     _____

     _____

   b. What is the key difference?

     _____

     _____

     _____

     _____

     _____

6. What are the various theories about the cause of hypochondriasis? (page 503)

_____

_____

_____

_____

_____

a. What conclusions can you draw from the existence of these competing theories?

_____

_____

_____

_____

_____

b. In terms of your own understanding of hypochondriasis and as a basis for treating these clients in your nursing practice, what theory do you personally embrace?

_____

_____

_____

_____

_____

7. What can a nurse do to help a person suffering from hypochondriasis? (pages 503–504)

_____

_____

_____

_____

_____

8. Conversion Disorder is one of the most puzzling and unimaginable of all the psychiatric disorders, and one of the hardest to treat. In your view, should nurses be confrontational toward clients with Conversion Disorder? Why or why not? (pages 504–506)

_____

_____

_____

_____

_____

9. Think about whether you believe the condition now known as Dissociative Identity Disorder (DID; formerly Multiple Personality Disorder) actually exists. (pages 509–510)

   a. Cite evidence and arguments for your view.

   _____

   _____

   _____

   _____

   _____

   b. Differentiate between schizophrenia and the disorder identified as Dissociative Identity Disorder.

   _____

   _____

   _____

   _____

   _____

10. Clients with somatoform disorders frequently become hostile when nurses question them about their symptoms, their past medical history, and stressors in their lives. Yet, these areas often produce the best assessment data. (page 513)

    a. Write five assessment questions you could use to assess a client with a suspected somatoform disorder, wording them in a way that is likely to elicit the best information.

    _____

    _____

    _____

    _____

    _____

b. List nursing diagnoses you think would be used frequently in caring for clients with somatoform disorders.

_____

_____

_____

_____

_____

SELF-ASSESSMENT QUIZ

1. People with alcoholism who experience blackouts should be diagnosed with which of the following? (page 508)

    a. Hypochondriasis

    b. Dissociative Amnesia Disorder

    c. Dependent Personality Disorder

    d. Generalized Anxiety Disorder

2. Individuals with Conversion Disorder (page 506)

    a. show a surprising indifference to their physical symptoms.

    b. express concern over physical ailments.

    c. disguise physical symptoms from the health care provider.

    d. lie about their physical symptoms.

3. Individuals with hypochondriasis (page 502)

    a. fake having a serious mental illness.

    b. fake having a serious physical illness.

    c. believe that they have a serious physical illness.

    d. believe that they have a major psychiatric illness.

4. Which treatment approaches are most effective in the treatment of hypochondriasis and Somatoform Disorders? (page 504)

    a. Psychotherapy and antipsychotics

    b. Cognitive therapy and antidepressants

    c. Reality therapy and antidepressants

    d. Behavioral therapy and antipsychotics

5. Which substance when found in the blood can help distinguish pseudoseizures from true epileptic convulsions? (page 506)

    a. Prolactin

    b. Dilantin

    c. Phenobarbital

    d. Cogentin

6. Of the classes of disorders discussed in this chapter, name one that does not fit into the DSM-IV-TR with the others. (page 496)

    a. Somatization Disorder

    b. Hypochondriasis

    c. Conversion Disorder

    d. Factitious Disorder

7. Which of the following is *not* true regarding the incidence of Somatization Disorder? (pages 500–501)

    a. It tends to show up in families in which another family member is diagnosed with Antisocial Personality Disorder.

    b. The disorder is predominantly associated with women.

    c. The disorder usually develops later in life.

    d. The disorder is comparatively rare.

8. Some of the long-used but unproven approaches to treating Conversion Disorder include all of the following except (page 506)

    a. hypnosis.

    b. faith healing or miracle cures.

    c. forced labor.

    d. exorcism.

9. When caring for a client with a Factitious Disorder, it is most helpful to keep the following in mind: (pages 510–511)

    a. Nurses should support one another when frustrated by clients with Factitious Disorder.

    b. Clients with Factitious Disorder are overutilizing an already overburdened health care system.

    c. Clients with Factitious Disorder take advantage of a nurse's normal caring and compassion when they fake health problems.

    d. Clients with Factitious Disorder are mentally ill and in need of appropriate psychiatric care.

    e. a and d

    f. a and c

10. Which of the following statements is true about Munchausen's Syndrome by Proxy? (page 507)

    a. It is a somatoform disorder, not a Factitious Disorder.

    b. Its victims are frequently the elderly.

    c. It is a form of child abuse reportable to Children's Protective Services.

    d. The father is usually the one with the mental illness.

Chapter 20

THE CLIENT WITH DISORDERS OF SELF-REGULATION: SLEEP DISORDERS, EATING DISORDERS, AND SEXUAL DISORDERS

The purpose of this chapter is to explore the basic human functions of sleeping, eating, and sexual activity normally associated with good mental health, and familiarize yourself with some of the more common disorders that interfere with the healthy exercise of these functions.

READING ASSIGNMENT

Please read Chapter 20, "The Client with Disorders of Self-Regulation: Sleep Disorders, Eating Disorders, and Sexual Disorders," pages 526–571.

KEY TERMS

Write definitions for the following terms in your own words. Compare your definitions with those given in the text.

Anorexia Nervosa _____

_____

Breathing-Related Sleep Disorders _____

_____

Bulimia Nervosa _____

_____

Cataplexy _____

_____

Dyssomnia _____

_____

Exhibitionism _____

_____

Fetishism _____

_____

Frotteurism _____

_____

Gender Dysphoria _____

_____

Gender Identity _____

_____

Gender Identity Disorder _____

_____

Gender Role _____

_____

Hypoactive Sexual Desire Disorder _____

_____

Insomnia _____

_____

Narcolepsy _____

_____

Nightmare _____

_____

Normal Sexual Behavior _____

_____

Paraphilia _____

_____

Parasomnia _____

_____

Pedophilia _____

_____

Primary Hypersomnia _____

_____

Primary Insomnia _____

_____

Restless Legs Syndrome (RLS) _____

_____

Sexual Dysfunction _____

_____

Sexual Masochism _____

_____

Sexual Sadism_____

_____

Sleep Hygiene _____

_____

Sleep Latency _____

_____

Sleep Paralysis _____

_____

Sleep Terrors _____

_____

Sleepwalking _____

_____

Transvestic Fetishism _____

_____

Voyeurism _____

_____

EXERCISES AND ACTIVITIES

1. You are no doubt familiar with the biological concept of homeostasis. The lifestyle concept equivalent is "balance." (page 529)

    a. Explain how the disorders discussed in this chapter are related to homeostasis and balance.

    _____

    _____

    _____

    _____

    _____

    b. Explain how the disorders discussed in this chapter relate to health, healthiness, and healthy lifestyles.

    _____

    _____

    _____

    _____

    _____

2. List the factors that can interfere with normal sleep. (page 529)

    _____

    _____

    _____

    _____

    _____

3. How would you counsel a person with Primary Insomnia—insomnia with no apparent external cause—to improve sleep hygiene? (pages 529-532)

_____

_____

_____

_____

_____

4. What has been the record of effectiveness of medications for insomnia? What is a good treatment alternative to medications for insomnia? (page 531)

_____

_____

_____

_____

_____

5. How would you counsel an adolescent to promote a healthy body image? (page 543)

_____

_____

_____

_____

_____

6. Describe the negative physical and physiological consequences associated with Anorexia Nervosa. (pages 544-546)

_____

_____

_____

_____

_____

7. Anorexia Nervosa appears to have puzzling origins. (page 545)

   a. What explanations exist for the psychological cause(s) of Anorexia Nervosa?

   _____

   _____

   _____

   _____

   _____

   b. Based on your study of the theories involved, what do you think is the cause of Anorexia Nervosa?

   _____

   _____

   _____

   _____

   _____

8. What are the three categories of sexual function disorders, and what are the differences among them? (page 553)

   _____

   _____

   _____

   _____

   _____

9. What strategies would you use to make a client feel comfortable and forthcoming when you are taking a sexual history as part of an overall health assessment? (page 553)

   _____

   _____

   _____

   _____

   _____

10. After reading this chapter, what do you consider to be the realm of "normal" sexual activity?

_____

_____

_____

_____

_____

SELF-ASSESSMENT QUIZ

1. Benzodiazepines are frequently prescribed for parasomnia to address which of the following? (page 536)

   a. Sleepwalking

   b. Sleep terrors

   c. Bedwetting

   d. Nightmares

2. Prazosin has been used to treat (page 536)

   a. sleepwalking.

   b. sleep terrors.

   c. bedwetting.

   d. nightmares.

3. Kunert, King, and Kolkhorst's 2007 study, "Fatigue and Sleep Quality and Nurses," revealed which of the following? (page 534)

   a. Nurses with less than 9 years of experience developed major sleep disturbances.

   b. Nurses with more than 20 years of experience perceived less fatigue and better sleep quality.

   c. Night-shift nurses reported greater daytime dysfunction than day-shift nurses.

   d. There were no differences in fatigue and sleep quality between day-shift and night-shift nurses.

4. Which of the following statements regarding Restless Legs Syndrome (RLS) is true? (page 535)

    a. Restless Legs Syndrome (RLS) affects 30% of the population.

    b. Restless Legs Syndrome (RLS) is more common in men.

    c. People with Restless Legs Syndrome (RLS) describe uncomfortable sensations in their legs.

    d. There is no genetic linkage with Restless Legs Syndrome (RLS).

5. Which of the following is a screening questionnaire for bulimia? (page 543)

    a. MMSE

    b. SCOFF

    c. FATFIND

    d. BRS

6. Which of the following statements about normal sleep is true? (pages 528-529)

    a. Although sleep deprivation causes people to feel unwell, there are no known serious adverse physiological consequences of sleep deprivation in an otherwise healthy person.

    b. There may be five stages of normal sleep, but the average person rarely goes through all five in a single night.

    c. It is a myth that sleep patterns change in old age.

    d. Scientists are on the verge of discovering all the secrets of sleep.

7. All of the following are primarily sleep disorders of children and adolescents, rather than adults, except (pages 534-535)

    a. narcolepsy.

    b. night terrors.

    c. sleepwalking.

    d. nightmares.

    e. a and b.

    f. a and c.

    g. a and d.

8. All of the following are disorders of sexual functioning except (pages 553–555)

    a. sadism.

    b. Hypoactive Sexual Desire Disorder.

    c. premature ejaculation.

    d. erectile disorder.

9. All of the following are widely recognized paraphilias except (page 556)

    a. voyeurism.

    b. pedophilia.

    c. fraterphilia.

    d. exhibitionism.

10. None of the following are recognized in the DSM-IV-TR as disorders except (page 539)

    a. Gender Identity Disorder.

    b. heterosexuality.

    c. Hyperactive Sexual Desire Disorder.

    d. homosexuality.

11. In developing a care plan for a client with a paraphilia, the nurse would include which of the following interventions?

    a. Long-term therapy and residential treatment

    b. Short-term therapy and residential treatment

    c. Alternative medicines and long-term treatment

    d. Medications and short-term treatment

Chapter 21

THE PHYSICALLY ILL CLIENT EXPERIENCING EMOTIONAL DISTRESS

The purpose of this chapter is to reinforce the point that virtually every person facing a serious physical disease experiences emotional stress, which can lead to symptoms of mental illness. Understanding the connections between the body and the mind is key to developing appropriate nursing care. The skills of psychiatric nursing are indispensable to the effective practice of nursing in virtually all settings.

READING ASSIGNMENT

Please read Chapter 21, "The Physically Ill Client Experiencing Emotional Distress," pages 575–598.

KEY TERMS

Write definitions for the following terms in your own words. Compare your definitions with those given in the text.

Mind Modulation _____

_____

Psychiatric Consultation-Liaison Nursing _____

_____

EXERCISES AND ACTIVITIES

1. State your beliefs about the body-mind connection. (pages 576–577)

   _____

   _____

   _____

   _____

   _____

2. How does the DSM-IV-TR handle the connection between serious physical illnesses and major mental illnesses? (page 577)

_____

_____

_____

_____

_____

3. Read Reflective Thinking 21-2 about reactions to very ill clients on page 580. If you found that your personal feelings interfered with your ability to effectively care for a particular client, what measures would you pursue to deal with the situation?

_____

_____

_____

_____

_____

4. Read the story of Dr. Lear's heart attack on pages 581–582.

    a. What efforts did Dr. Lear make to maintain control over his situation?

    _____

    _____

    _____

    _____

    _____

    b. Were these efforts to maintain control therapeutic, destructive, or both?

    _____

    _____

    _____

    _____

    _____

c. What interventions by others did Dr. Lear find comforting?

_____

_____

_____

_____

_____

d. Did these interventions interfere with his need to maintain control over his situation?

_____

_____

_____

_____

_____

5. What interventions can a nurse perform to treat a family member who has the nursing diagnosis of caregiver role strain?

_____

_____

_____

_____

_____

6. Write a job description for a liaison psychiatric nurse. (pages 591–592)

_____

_____

_____

_____

_____

7. Study Table 21-1 on page 593.

   a. Do you agree with the correlations suggested between the nursing process and Erickson's theory?

   _____

   _____

   _____

   _____

   _____

   b. Consulting the list of NANDA nursing diagnoses in Appendix B (page 940), make a list of nursing diagnoses that would be commonly used for a client having difficulty adapting to a severe physical illness.

   _____

   _____

   _____

   _____

   _____

8. Name five psychiatric disorders or psychosocial nursing diagnoses that were associated with the outbreak of severe acute respiratory syndrome (SARS) in China.

   _____

   _____

   _____

   _____

   _____

9. Look up *stress* in your medical surgical or pathophysiology textbook. What evidence does it cite to support an explanation of stress (General Adaptation Syndrome) based on the new science of psychoneuroimmunology? Record the highlights here.

   _____

   _____

   _____

   _____

   _____

10. Nurses, it is said, are at the forefront in understanding and making use of the body-mind connection. Why do you think this is a significant domain for nurses?

_____

_____

_____

_____

_____

SELF-ASSESSMENT QUIZ

1. A client who was recently diagnosed with breast cancer is scheduled for a mastectomy. When developing the plan for client care, an appropriate outcome would be which of the following? (pages 578–580)

    a. The client expresses feeling overwhelmed by the demands of the treatment.

    b. The nurse will set goals for the client that are health related.

    c. The client will be able to cope effectively with her illness.

    d. The nurse will provide support and caring during the client's surgery.

2. The nurse caring for clients diagnosed with cancer understands which of the following? (pages 578–580)

    a. Individuals must call on adaptive strengths when facing life-threatening illnesses.

    b. There is a major difference between having a physical illness and having a mental health illness.

    c. The diagnosis of cancer is always directly related to the client's poor lifestyle choices.

    d. Cancer is hereditary and cannot be prevented.

3. When caring for a client with cancer, an appropriate question to ask for a spiritual assessment would be which of the following? (page 581)

    a. "Do you belong to any formal religious group?"

    b. "Do you attend church on a regular basis?"

    c. "How has your cancer influenced your faith or beliefs?"

    d. "What information would you like to have about your cancer and the treatment?"

4. When caring for a client experiencing guilt regarding a diagnosis of cancer, which nursing intervention is most therapeutic? (pages 583–584)

    a. Assure the client that many forms of cancer are curable.

    b. Accept the client where she is and practice the art of unconditional acceptance.

    c. Tell the client that constantly talking about the cancer will not change the outcome.

    d. Understand that guilt is a defense mechanism used to avoid responsibility.

5. Nurses involved in treating chronic pain often face the social expectation that medications should not be given to clients experiencing pain related to which of the following? (page 587)

    a. Cancer

    b. Rheumatoid arthritis

    c. Heart disease

    d. Cocaine withdrawal

6. All of the following are measures that nurses can use to establish trust except

    a. setting aside time to spend with clients.

    b. keeping appointments with clients.

    c. reading each client's chart.

    d. keeping promises made to clients.

7. *Mind modulation* refers to (pages 593–594)

    a. the mechanism with which the body transforms thoughts, emotions, attitudes, and images into neurohormonal messenger molecules.

    b. the use of sound waves to affect brain waves.

    c. a nursing theory that helps clients cope with stress.

    d. psychosurgery.

8. Mr. Davies may have died as a result of his mental illness not being treated after his second heart attack. His DSM-IV-TR diagnosis should have been (page 577)

   a. mood disorder due to a general medical condition.

   b. Major Depressive Disorder as an Axis I diagnosis without any Axis III diagnosis.

   c. Major Depressive Disorder as an Axis I diagnosis with an Axis III diagnosis of diseases of the circulatory system (myocardial infarction).

   d. hopelessness.

9. Which of the following measures is *not* an example of offering a client "unconditional acceptance"? (pages 592–594)

   a. Helping clients identify personal strengths

   b. Planning to spend unstructured time with clients

   c. Pointing out that better health habits might have prevented the current illness

   d. Providing interventions that enhance comfort

10. Emily Dickinson wrote, "Hope is the thing with feathers." In his book *Without Feathers*, Woody Allen noted that hopelessness can be fatal. Nurses can foster the healing power of hope in a client experiencing hopelessness by all of the following except (pages 592–594)

    a. forming a caring relationship with the client.

    b. reassuring the client that everything will turn out all right.

    c. helping the client regain control over health-related decision making.

    d. helping the client make lifestyle adaptations that will help facilitate recovery or adapt to the client's changing health state.

Chapter 22

FORGOTTEN POPULATIONS:
THE HOMELESS AND THE INCARCERATED

The purpose of this chapter is to focus on two demographic groups with high rates of mental illness, the homeless and the incarcerated. While prisoners usually have access to excellent health care services, homeless people generally do not.

READING ASSIGNMENT

Please read Chapter 22, "Forgotten Populations: The Homeless and the Incarcerated," pages 600–618.

KEY TERMS

Write definitions for the following terms in your own words. Compare your definitions with those given in the text.

Deinstitutionalization _____

_____

Homelessness_____

_____

Incarcerated _____

_____

NIMBY Syndrome _____

_____

EXERCISES AND ACTIVITIES

1. Read the chapter opening on page 600.

    a. Write down your personal responses to the homeless and to the incarcerated.

    _____

    _____

    _____

    _____

    _____

    b. Regardless of your personal views, which to some extent reflect your values, is there anything that would hold you back from providing members of these groups the same quality of nursing care you would provide to anyone else?

    _____

    _____

    _____

    _____

    _____

2. Name four factors that have contributed to the increase in homelessness since 1975. (page 604)

    _____

    _____

    _____

    _____

    _____

3. If you are old enough to have this perspective, do you personally agree that homelessness has increased considerably since 1975, compared to years earlier? One of the culprits is the deinstitutionalization of the chronically mentally ill. Deinstitutionalization had been going on since the 1950s, however; what made the problem of homelessness so much worse after 1975?

4. Name the major health problems of homeless people. (pages 604–606)

5. Consulting the list of NANDA nursing diagnoses in Appendix B on page 940, list those nursing diagnoses that would be likely to have the most frequent application to the homeless.

6. What are the major health problems faced by people in prison? (pages 610–613)

7. With wars, refugees, terrorism, and asylum-seeking immigration on the rise, American nurses are more likely to be called upon to provide treatment to victims of torture. What adverse mental health outcomes are prevalent among survivors of politically driven torture? (page 614)

_____

_____

_____

_____

_____

8. What conditions present the greatest risk of suicide among the incarcerated? (page 612)

_____

_____

_____

_____

_____

9. In what ways can nurses be effective advocates for the homeless and the incarcerated? (pages 614–615)

_____

_____

_____

_____

_____

10. Identify the homeless shelter closest to where you live. Volunteer at the shelter to learn more about the extent of the homeless problem in your community and the specific factors and problems affecting your local homeless population.

SELF-ASSESSMENT QUIZ

1. Which of the following is a true statement? (page 604)

    a. The longer people stay homeless, the more difficult it is to remove them from that subculture.

    b. Early interventions have no impact on reducing the length of homelessness.

    c. Homelessness is directly related to the inability to make positive life choices.

    d. Very few women and children are among the homeless population.

2. One study documented that what percentage of individuals discharged from a large public hospital in the United States were homeless at the time of discharge? (page 608)

    a. 10.1%

    b. 25.6%

    c. 32.3%

    d. 40.5%

3. Psychosis, depression, and which other disorders are found more commonly among the imprisoned than in the general population? (page 611)

    a. Anxiety disorders

    b. Somatoform disorders

    c. Personality disorders

    d. Eating disorders

4. In a study describing the perceptions of female prisoners regarding their health and health care needs, the researcher found that the subjects did not seek treatment for serious problems because of all of the following except (page 612)

    a. lack of privacy.

    b. long waiting times.

    c. lack of dignity.

    d. most health providers were female.

Chapter 23

THE CHILD

The purpose of this chapter is to review the major psychiatric disorders of childhood which, like the medical diseases of childhood, differ significantly in type and character from adult disorders. Inasmuch as children cannot choose their living circumstances in the way adults can, they present special challenges to the mental health community, and their care cannot always be separated from the mental health care of their caregivers.

READING ASSIGNMENT

Please read Chapter 23, "The Child," pages 620–652.

KEY TERMS

Write definitions for the following terms in your own words. Compare your definitions with those given in the text.

Asperger's Syndrome _____

_____

Autism _____

_____

Conduct Disorder _____

_____

Dysthymia _____

_____

Oppositional Defiant Disorder _____

_____

Reactive Depression _____

_____

Separation Anxiety _____

_____

Social Phobia _____

_____

EXERCISES AND ACTIVITIES

1. Most adults have positive feelings toward children who are loveable and well behaved. In mental health settings, however, you will encounter children who are less approachable and may exhibit unlikable behavior. State in your own words your usual response to children like this.

   _____

   _____

   _____

   _____

   _____

2. What are the DSM-IV-TR diagnostic criteria for Attention-Deficit Hyperactivity Disorder (ADHD)? Think in terms of number of symptoms, variety of settings, age of onset, and functional impairment. (page 624)

   _____

   _____

   _____

   _____

   _____

3. Treatment of ADHD is termed *multi-modal*. Describe a complete treatment program for a child with ADHD. (page 626)

   _____

   _____

   _____

   _____

   _____

4. Think about what you learned about the major mood disorders in Chapter 14, Major Depressive Disorder, Dysthymic Disorder, and Bipolar Disorder. (pages 627-631)

   a. What differences are seen, if any, when these disorders are manifested in children?

   _____

   _____

   _____

   _____

   _____

   _____

   b. What differences in efficacy are seen, if any, in the treatments available for adults and children—particularly young children—for major mood disorders?

   _____

   _____

   _____

   _____

   _____

5. What factors would you include in assessing the seriousness of a child's suicidal ideation or behavior? (pages 627-628)

   _____

   _____

   _____

   _____

   _____

6. Separation anxiety is quite normal for an infant or toddler. What characteristics make it pathological? (pages 631-632)

   _____

   _____

   _____

   _____

   _____

7. For the following anxiety disorders, identify the ones found commonly only in childhood with a "C," and those found in both children and adults with an "A." Indicate the forms of effective treatment. (pages 623, 626, 631–632)

	Drug Therapy	Other Tx
Attention-Deficit Hyperactivity Disorder		
Generalized Anxiety Disorder		
Separation Anxiety		
Social Phobia		
Obsessive-Compulsive Disorder		

8. Differentiate Asperger's Syndrome from autism. What treatments, if any, seem efficacious? (pages 633–636)

_____

_____

_____

_____

_____

9. A continuum of severity, from less disruptive to more disruptive, exists among Oppositional Defiant Disorder (ODD), Conduct Disorder, and Antisocial Personality Disorder. (page 636)

a. How would you differentiate among these disorders?

_____

_____

_____

_____

_____

b. What risk factors may contribute to these developmental disorders?

_____

_____

_____

_____

_____

c. What treatment options seem viable for each of these disruptive disorders?

_____

_____

_____

_____

_____

10. In your own words, state the current thinking on treating childhood depression and anxiety with SSRIs.

_____

_____

_____

_____

_____

11. In your own words, discuss the primary reason children with ADHD are sometimes treated with the patch version of methylphenidate instead of an oral version. (page 627)

_____

_____

_____

_____

_____

SELF-ASSESSMENT QUIZ

1. Closed head injury in children may result in which of the following? (page 626)

a. Asperger's Syndrome

b. Reactive Depression

c. Attention-Deficit Hyperactivity Disorder (ADHD)

d. Obsessive-Compulsive Disorder

2. The putamen part of the basal ganglia of the brain is involved in (page 626)

    a. movement.

    b. vision.

    c. learning.

    d. digestion.

3. Atomoxetine now carries an FDA warning regarding the development of suicidal ideations and which other condition? (page 626)

    a. Renal impairment

    b. Cardiac arrhythmias

    c. Sleep disturbances

    d. Liver toxicity

4. What is the most common form of mood disorder in children? (page 628)

    a. Dysthymia

    b. Reactive Depression

    c. Major Depressive Disorder

    d. Bipolar Disorder

5. Which group of children has the highest rate of depression? (page 630)

    a. American Indians

    b. African Americans

    c. Caucasians

    d. Pacific Islanders

6. Which of the following statements shows how the manic phase of Bipolar Disorder in children is differentiated from ADHD? (page 630)

    a. Hyperactive behavior is episodic or cyclical.

    b. ADHD responds to Ritalin.

    c. Bipolar Disorder does not occur until late adolescence.

    d. Children with Bipolar Disorder do not allow their behavior to get them in trouble as children with ADHD do.

7. Which of the following is *not* a normal expression of Separation Anxiety? (page 631)

   a. A 3-year-old has to stay overnight at the home of a family friend due to an emergency.

   b. A 6-year-old has experienced several traumatic events.

   c. A preteen is exceptionally shy.

   d. A 9-year-old won't go to camp or sleep at a friend's house.

8. Which of the following criteria is appropriate for considering a diagnosis of Conduct Disorder? (page 637)

   a. Isolated acts of misbehavior

   b. Antisocial behavior beyond what would be expected in normal growth and development

   c. Socioeconomic status

   d. School performance

9. The brains of children with autism seem to differ from the brains of normal children in all these ways except (pages 634–635)

   a. only one hemisphere grows to maturity.

   b. serotonin synthesis is decreased.

   c. brains of autistic children often start out undersized but then experience rapid growth.

   d. the hox1 may be abnormal.

10. All of the following are risk factors for childhood emotional disorders except (page 638)

   a. physical disability of the child.

   b. poverty.

   c. caregiver psychopathology.

   d. divorce.

11. Play therapy is used for all the following therapeutic purposes except (pages 641–642)

    a. caregiver training.

    b. exploring relationships.

    c. as a substitute for verbal interaction.

    d. attempting new solutions to problems.

Chapter 24

THE ADOLESCENT

The purpose of this chapter is to understand the most turbulent time of human development, the transition from childhood to adulthood known as adolescence. You should become familiar with the mental health disorders associated with this period and be able to differentiate the mental health problems of adolescence from the normal turbulence of adolescence.

READING ASSIGNMENT

Please read Chapter 24, "The Adolescent," pages 654–681.

KEY TERMS

Write definitions for the following terms in your own words. Compare your definitions with those given in the text.

Foreclosure _____

_____

Gender Identity _____

_____

Gender Role _____

_____

Identity Achievement _____

_____

Identity Diffusion _____

_____

Identity Formation _____

_____

Identity Status _____

_____

Moratorium _____

_____

Presence _____

_____

Self-Awareness _____

_____

Self-Efficacy _____

_____

Sexual Orientation _____

_____

Social Competence _____

_____

Suicidal Ideation _____

_____

Transgender _____

_____

EXERCISES AND ACTIVITIES

1. Read the chapter opening on page 656.

   a. What problems did you experience in adolescence?

   _____

   _____

   _____

   _____

   _____

   b. Do you think it is harder to go through adolescence today than it was during your adolescent years? In what ways?

   _____

   _____

   _____

   _____

   _____

c. How did your current sense of personal identity develop during your adolescence? Has it changed since? In what ways?

_____

_____

_____

_____

_____

2. Adolescence is characterized by cognitive changes and decision making that may be characterized by lack of impulse control, risk taking, and lack of regard for long-term consequences. List problems that often result from this feature of adolescence.

_____

_____

_____

_____

_____

3. Identify the three stages of adolescence; include descriptors. (pages 656–657)

_____

_____

_____

_____

_____

4. Review Table 24-1, "Four Statuses Identity Statuses," on page 660.

a. Which status best reflects your own adolescence?

_____

_____

_____

_____

_____

b. Can you visualize adolescents you have known who fit into the other statuses?

_____

_____

_____

_____

_____

5. Middle adolescents often conform to their peers in their search for what's "normal." How would you counsel such an adolescent in terms of explaining what's normal for the age group?

_____

_____

_____

_____

_____

6. Summarize the risk factors associated with adolescent suicide. (pages 663–667)

_____

_____

_____

_____

_____

7. List some strategies for talking with an adolescent therapeutically about sex. (page 667)

_____

_____

_____

_____

_____

8. How would you teach an adolescent about how to prevent AIDS and other STDs?

_____

_____

_____

_____

_____

9. Test your knowledge of adolescent culture by making a list of current expressions, musicians, and popular culture icons currently favored by adolescents.

_____

_____

_____

_____

_____

10. Explain in your own words what *humanistic nursing* is. (pages 686–687)

_____

_____

_____

_____

_____

11. What measures could you use to establish rapport with an adolescent whose racial or ethnic identity is different from your own?

_____

_____

_____

_____

_____

12. Match the stage of adolescent development with the appropriate description. (page 660)

    a. Foreclosure   _____ Identity decision made before options explored

    b. Identity achievement   _____ Identity decision delayed until options explored

    c. Identity diffusion   _____ Identity decision avoided

    d. Moratorium   _____ Identity decision made after options explored

SELF-ASSESSMENT QUIZ

1. According to the CDC (2008), how many children and adolescents between the ages of 9 and 17 had a diagnosable behavioral or emotional health problem? (pages 662-663)

    a. 1 in 5

    b. 1 in 10

    c. 1 in 15

    d. 1 in 20

2. Which of the following best defines *gender role*? (page 664)

    a. Individual's subjective or private experience of gender

    b. Individual's expression of attraction to members of the opposite or the same sex

    c. Individual's confusion over sex assignment at birth

    d. Public recognition of an individual's sexual assignment

3. What percentage of children ages 7-12 run away from home each year? (page 666)

    a. 2%

    b. 6%

    c. 12%

    d. 15%

4. According to Erikson's theory of growth and development, the central developmental task of adolescence is (page 659)

    a. trust vs. mistrust.

    b. intimacy vs. isolation.

    c. identity vs. role confusion.

    d. integrity vs. stagnation.

5. Recent developments in neuroimaging and genetics suggest that the development of the brain is (page 657)

    a. in its beginning stage by adolescence.

    b. complete by the beginning of adolescence.

    c. complete by the end of adolescence.

    d. not complete by the end of adolescence.

6. Social competence is a concept characterized by (page 661)

    a. choosing friends wisely.

    b. having good manners.

    c. decoding, interpreting, and responding to social cues.

    d. being able to move easily among social classes.

7. All of the following psychiatric disorders can originate in adolescence except (pages 662–664)

    a. schizophrenia.

    b. autism.

    c. Conduct Disorder.

    d. anorexia nervosa.

8. Warning signs of potential adolescent suicide include (page 666)

    a. increased risk taking, interest in shaving, and upcoming important dates.

    b. previous suicidal gestures, giving away possessions, and getting an after-school job.

    c. expression of wish to die, stated feelings of sadness or despair, and sudden deterioration of behavior or appearance and hygiene.

    d. alienating behavior, preoccupation with death or dying, and mild disappointment.

9. Which of the following assessment findings would make a nurse feel concerned about the mental health of an adolescent client? (page 672)

    a. Inability to concentrate on tasks at hand; numbness or lack of affect; inability to maintain eye contact

    b. Inability to tolerate young children; constant wearing of earphones; using vulgar or provocative language

    c. Constant fidgeting; anger and hostility; admiration for rock stars

    d. Inability to maintain eye contact; rolls eyes when mother speaks; wants to drive the family car

10. Statistically, adolescents are at the greatest risk for developing mental health problems if they are (page 666)

    a. from single-caregiver families in which the caregiver has a history of mental problems.

    b. from middle-class homes.

    c. smoking cigarettes before age 12.

    d. never going to learn to drive.

11. Studies show that the main factor that protects adolescents best from dangerous and risky behavior is (page 667)

    a. good genes.

    b. connectedness with parents and school.

    c. desire for attention.

    d. character traits such as will power.

Chapter 25

THE ELDERLY

The purpose of this chapter is to gain an appreciation for the unique mental health needs and problems experienced by the elderly. It also includes a discussion of the needs of those who are charged with caring for the elderly.

READING ASSIGNMENT

Please read Chapter 25, "The Elderly," pages 682–721.

KEY TERMS

Write definitions for the following terms in your own words. Compare your definitions with those given in the text.

Agnosia _____

_____

Aphasia _____

_____

Apraxia _____

_____

Catastrophic Reaction _____

_____

Cognition _____

_____

Confabulation _____

_____

Confusion _____

_____

Delirium _____

_____

Dementia _____

_____

Mutuality _____

_____

EXERCISES AND ACTIVITIES

1. Many older people who become victims of dementia actually recognize the early signs of failing memory and coming dysfunction. (page 686)

    a. If you recognized these early symptoms in yourself, what treatment would you seek?

    _____

    _____

    _____

    _____

    _____

    b. What precautions would you take, or what alterations would you make in your daily functioning?

    _____

    _____

    _____

    _____

    _____

    c. What legal, financial, and family decisions would you make?

    _____

    _____

    _____

    _____

    _____

2. Identify the four types of cognitive disorders in the elderly and define them. (page 687)

_____

_____

_____

_____

_____

3. Differentiate among delirium, confusion, and acute confusional states. What is the terminology appropriate for health care professionals? (pages 687–689)

_____

_____

_____

_____

_____

4. Define *dignity* in your own words.

_____

_____

_____

_____

a. What measures could you implement to help preserve the dignity of a client who was being placed in a nursing home against the client's wishes?

_____

_____

_____

_____

b. What measures could you implement to help preserve the dignity of a client who needed assistance with dressing, eating, toileting, or walking?

_____

_____

_____

_____

_____

c. What measures could you implement to help preserve the dignity of a client who had been placed in restraints?

_____

_____

_____

_____

_____

d. The authors suggest several characteristics of a more progressive nursing home environment. What do they suggest? Could you add ideas of your own?

_____

_____

_____

_____

_____

5. Review the Geriatric Depression Scale on page 697. What score is indicative of depression?

_____

_____

_____

_____

_____

6. Name the four subtypes of depression and differentiate them from one another. (pages 694–695)

_____

_____

_____

_____

_____

7. Read the poem "Survived by His Wife" on page 695. Explain why the author compares the possessions of the dead husband to "frames of stolen paintings left behind."

_____

_____

_____

_____

_____

8. Define "self-transcendence" and its relationship to risk for suicide. (page 699)

_____

_____

_____

_____

_____

9. Research is making progress in helping to explain the origins and pathophysiology of Alzheimer's Disease. (pages 702–703)

    a. Differentiate between Early-Onset and Late-Onset Alzheimer's Disease. What seems to be the cause of the Early-Onset variety?

    _____

    _____

    _____

    _____

    _____

b. Two defining findings associated with Alzheimer's Disease are beta-amyloid plaques and neurofibrillary tangles. Why do these processes seem to be so debilitating? What seems to cause them?

_____

_____

_____

_____

_____

c. What treatments may contribute to slowing down the course of Alzheimer's Disease?

_____

_____

_____

_____

_____

d. What treatments may delay the onset of or prevent Alzheimer's Disease?

_____

_____

_____

_____

_____

e. What seems to be the effect of brain infarction on Alzheimer's Disease?

_____

_____

_____

_____

_____

10. Write a script of a conversation with an older person with dementia, identifying when the client is confabulating. (page 705)

_____

_____

_____

_____

_____

SELF-ASSESSMENT QUIZ

1. Elders with dementia are at increased risk for which of the following? (page 688)

    a. Anxiety

    b. Delirium

    c. Schizophrenia

    d. Narcolepsy

2. When using the acronym IWATCH to identify the pathologies that may cause delirium, the nurse recognizes that the "W" represents (page 688)

    a. water intoxication related to fluid overload.

    b. wandering behaviors associated with sleep disturbances.

    c. withdrawal from alcohol, barbiturates, or sedatives.

    d. widow or widower marital status.

3. Which of the following assessment tools for ACS/Delirium would be used to identify clients "at risk"? (page 689)

    a. Delirium Rating Scale (DRS)

    b. Memorial Delirium Scale

    c. Mini-Mental State Exam (MMSE)

    d. NEECHAM Confessional Scale

4. Which of the following is the fastest-growing age group in the population? (page 684)

   a. Infants under 1 year of age

   b. Children and adolescents

   c. Adults between 55 and 70

   d. People over the age of 85

5. The anticholinergic side effect of tricyclic medications places the elderly client at risk for which of the following? (page 698)

   a. Falls

   b. Dehydration

   c. Cardiac arrhythmias

   d. Fluid and electrolyte imbalance

6. All of the following can cause dementia except (page 688)

   a. schizophrenia.

   b. syphilis.

   c. Parkinson's Disease.

   d. head injury.

7. All of the following are typical behaviors associated with dementia except (pages 718–721)

   a. paranoia.

   b. hypochondria.

   c. aggression.

   d. wandering.

8. The best strategy for understanding a client with aphasia would be to (page 707)

   a. ask the client to repeat himself until you understand.

   b. repeat something that sounds to you like what the client said.

   c. ask "yes" and "no" questions to clarify what the client wants.

   d. smile and reassure the client.

9. Nurses can help caregivers of clients with dementia in all the following ways except (pages 716–717)

   a. explaining the diagnosis honestly and frankly.

   b. encouraging the making of legal and financial decisions as soon as possible, with the participation of the client if possible.

   c. encouraging the client and caregiver to participate in insight-oriented therapy.

   d. making the caregiver aware of community resources.

10. Nurses can help caregivers to accept their decision to place a loved one in a nursing home by all of the following except (page 716)

   a. encouraging the caregiver to take a cruise or "do something for yourself for a change."

   b. helping the caregiver see any humor there may be in the situation.

   c. pointing out that the client will adapt to the nursing home over time.

   d. reminding the caregiver that the nursing home may be in a position to provide better care for the client than the client could have continued to get at home.

Chapter 26

VIOLENCE: AN ISSUE FOR PSYCHIATRIC MENTAL HEALTH NURSING

The purpose of this chapter is to focus on the care of victims of violence, our most serious social problem. Understanding the dynamics of relationships that spark violence helps to promote safety and health care. Victims of violence and abuse often require special health care. This chapter helps the psychiatric nurse to provide care needed by this large group of victims.

READING ASSIGNMENT

Please read Chapter 26, "Violence: An Issue for Psychiatric Mental Health Nursing," pages 722-761.

KEY TERMS

Write definitions for the following terms in your own words. Compare your definitions with those given in the text.

Battery _____

_____

Bullying _____

_____

Child Abuse _____

_____

Child Molestation_____

_____

Child Neglect _____

_____

Child Pornography_____

_____

Child Soldiers _____

_____

Domestic Violence _____

_____

Elder Abuse _____

_____

Elder Neglect _____

_____

Incest _____

_____

Intimate Partner Violence (IPV) _____

_____

Mental Injury _____

_____

Negligent Treatment _____

_____

Physical Injury _____

_____

Rape _____

_____

Refugee _____

_____

Sexual Abuse (Child) _____

_____

Sexual Abuse (Elder) _____

_____

Sexual Exploitation _____

_____

Stranger Violence _____

_____

Structural Violence _____

_____

Suicide _____

_____

Trafficking _____

_____

Violence _____

_____

EXERCISES AND ACTIVITIES

1. List the myths regarding rape that you are familiar with.

_____

_____

_____

_____

_____

2. Nurses are usually required to report domestic violence to the authorities when they become aware of it. When fulfilling this legal obligation, nurses should take what precautions to protect the survivor in the coming crisis? (page 747)

_____

_____

_____

_____

_____

3. Some victims of intimate partner violence (IPV) feel trapped and stay with their tormenter; others find the wherewithal to leave the abusive relationship. (pages 735–737)

   a. List the circumstances that can be helpful for an abused partner to seriously consider leaving the abuser.

   b. List the reasons many abused partners cannot bring themselves to leave their abusers.

   c. How would you counsel a battered partner who doesn't feel able to leave the batterer?

4. What information should be included in a child abuse report? (page 729)

5. Review Box 26-2,"Characteristics of Child Abuse and Neglect," on page 731. Design an assessment tool you could use to help identify children at risk for abuse.

_____

_____

_____

_____

_____

6. Explain how refugees may be the victims of violence. (pages 741–742)

   a. What are the primary health care needs of victims of human trafficking?

_____

_____

_____

_____

_____

   b. Explain how the nurse can assist victims of human trafficking.

_____

_____

_____

_____

_____

7. When mothers are exposed to intimate partner violence, their children are also at risk of developing behavioral problems. What kind of behavior should you look for in these children? What nursing interventions should you undertake on behalf of the children of abused or battered mothers? (pages 748–750)

_____

_____

_____

_____

8. What are some of the signs and symptoms that should prompt nurses to consider the possibility of intimate partner or domestic violence? (pages 735–738)

     _____

     _____

     _____

     _____

     _____

9. What are some examples of violence in the workplace? (page 738)

     _____

     _____

     _____

     _____

     _____

10. Were you ever in a situation when you felt a loss of control and another person had complete power and control over your personal safety and well-being? Try to reconstruct the kinds of feelings any client might feel in such a situation.

     _____

     _____

     _____

     _____

     _____

11. After reading Chapter 26, answer the following questions.

    a. Think about when you were in high school. What types of violence were you aware of in your own home, school, and/or community?

     _____

     _____

     _____

     _____

     _____

b. How were these issues of violence addressed?

_____

_____

_____

_____

_____

c. How did you feel when you heard about the violence?

_____

_____

_____

_____

_____

d. As a nurse, how would you plan to support the victims of the type of violence you stated above?

_____

_____

_____

_____

_____

e. Do you feel violence in the schools has increased or decreased since you graduated from high school?

_____

_____

_____

_____

_____

12. Choose any newspaper. How many acts of violence were reported in the first 10 pages of the newspaper?

_____

_____

_____

_____

_____

SELF-ASSESSMENT QUIZ

1. A woman is brought to the Emergency Department after being attacked and robbed. The nurse understands that what percentage of robberies of women is perpetrated by someone they know? (page 740)

   a. 10%

   b. 25%

   c. 50%

   d. 75%

2. Which individual is most likely to be involved with gangs? (page 740)

   a. 15-year-old Asian male from a middle-class family

   b. 16-year-old Hispanic male from a poor family

   c. 17-year-old African American girl from a poor family

   d. 18-year-old Caucasian male from a poor family

3. One of the most current approaches to studying abuse and violence is the (page 726)

   a. psychoanalytic approach.

   b. behavioral approach.

   c. ecological approach.

   d. humanistic approach.

4. A school nurse teaches a group of elementary students actions to take if they are bullied by another student. This is an example of which type of prevention? (page 749–750)

    a. Primary prevention

    b. Secondary prevention

    c. Tertiary prevention

    d. Quarterly prevention

5. A nurse has cared for a number of clients who were victims of abuse and violence. The nurse's approach is based on the belief that violent behavior is influenced by interactions among personal predisposition, relationships, community, and society. Which perspective of violence is the nurse using? (page 726)

    a. Ecological

    b. Psychoanalytic

    c. Interpersonal

    d. Behavioral

Chapter 27

PHARMACOLOGY IN PSYCHIATRIC CARE

The purpose of this chapter is to familiarize you with psychopharmacology and the pharmacological treatment of clients with psychiatric disorders. Drug therapy has become the dominant mode of treatment for many forms of mental illness, and it is an area of intensive research and rapid development. It is essential to understand the pharmacological action and nursing considerations associated with each major drug class and many widely used individual drugs. It is also important to know how to find drug information when you need it, and when you need to teach your clients about the medications they are taking.

READING ASSIGNMENT

Please read Chapter 27, "Pharmacology in Psychiatric Care," pages 764–803.

KEY TERMS

Write definitions for the following terms in your own words. Compare your definitions with those given in the text.

Akathisia _____

_____

Antipsychotic Drugs _____

_____

Blood-Brain Barrier _____

_____

Dystonia _____

_____

Half-Life_____

_____

Neuroleptic Malignant Syndrome_____

_____

Oculogyric Crisis _____

_____

Serotonergic Syndrome_____

_____

Tardive Dyskinesia _____

_____

Therapeutic Window_____

_____

EXERCISES AND ACTIVITIES

1. Name the two broad classes of antipsychotic drugs and differentiate between them. (pages 771–772)

   _____

   _____

   _____

   _____

   _____

2. Review the drug actions of antipsychotics on page 768.

   a. What are the two actions associated with antipsychotic drugs?

      _____

      _____

      _____

      _____

      _____

b. How are antipsychotics similar to and different from narcotics and sedatives?

_____

_____

_____

_____

_____

c. Characterize the benefits and drawbacks of risperidone.

_____

_____

_____

_____

_____

d. If haloperidol is less expensive than the atypical neuroleptics, why did the authors suggest that treatment with atypical neuroleptics might be less expensive overall?

_____

_____

_____

_____

_____

3. What are the main adverse effects resulting from use of antipsychotics? (pages 773-775)

_____

_____

_____

_____

_____

4. Name the four classes of drugs used to treat mood disorders. (page 776)

_____

_____

_____

_____

_____

5. When a client is given a tricyclic antidepressant, how long will it take for the client to feel relief from depression? (page 778)

_____

_____

_____

_____

_____

  a. What symptoms may improve before the depression itself improves?

_____

_____

_____

_____

_____

  b. What side effects should the nurse be alert to?

_____

_____

_____

_____

_____

6. What considerations should the clinician take into account when deciding what kind of antidepressant should be prescribed for a client with clinical depression? (pages 776–787)

_____

_____

_____

_____

_____

7. How would you counsel a client who is experiencing unpleasant side effects from antidepressants and wants to discontinue using them?

_____

_____

_____

_____

_____

8. Teaching clients about medications is an important nursing function. (pages 776–790)

   a. What teaching would you provide to a client who has been prescribed an MAO inhibitor?

_____

_____

_____

_____

   b. What teaching would you provide to a client who has been prescribed lithium?

_____

_____

_____

_____

9. Why are so many new antidepressants coming onto the market? What characterizes these new antidepressants? (pages 785–787)

_____

_____

_____

_____

_____

10. Briefly state the advantages of the following medications: (page 793)

a. Buspirone (BuSpar)

_____

_____

_____

_____

_____

b. Zolpidem (Ambien)

_____

_____

_____

_____

_____

c. Propranolol (Inderal)

_____

_____

_____

_____

_____

11. Why do people respond differently to the same drugs, and why do drugs cause different side effects—or no side effects at all—in different people?

_____

_____

_____

_____

_____

12. What are some of the potential adverse affects of antipsychotic medications used to treat the elderly? (page 774)

_____

_____

_____

_____

_____

SELF-ASSESSMENT QUIZ

1. Which new long-acting second-generation antipsychotic may require administration only every four weeks? (page 773)

    a. Risperidone

    b. Ziprasidone

    c. Iloperidone

    d. Clozapine

2. Which atypical antipsychotic has shown significantly more effectiveness than other atypical antipsychotics in use for treating refractory schizophrenia? (page 771)

    a. Clozapine (Clozaril)

    b. Olanzapine (Zyprexa)

    c. Quetiapine (Seroquel)

    d. Aripiprazole (Abilify)

3. Antipsychotic medications bind strongly to brain receptors for (page 768)

   a. serotonin.

   b. dopamine.

   c. epinephrine.

   d. norepinephrine.

4. A client is receiving Valium for anxiety. Which of the following is a major concern related to long-term use of this medication? (page 792)

   a. Tolerance

   b. Addiction

   c. Sensitization

   d. Physical dependence

5. Which of the following is a low-potency antipsychotic? (page 772)

   a. Thorazine

   b. Prolixin

   c. Haldol

   d. Stelazine

6. Disadvantages of current antipsychotic drugs include all of the following except which? (pages 769–771)

   a. They control symptoms, but they don't cure diseases.

   b. Many people with the most severe symptoms are not helped by the currently available drugs.

   c. The currently available drugs can cause devastating side effects.

   d. Many currently available antipsychotics are also used to treat other health problems.

7. It is believed that many psychotropic drugs are effective because (page 769)

   a. their molecules are too large to pass the blood-brain barrier.

   b. they bind to proteins.

   c. they bind to brain receptors for dopamine.

   d. they cannot modify neurotransmitters.

8. Which of the following is the safest antidepressant to prescribe to a pregnant or lactating woman? (page 784)

    a. No antidepressant should ever be prescribed to a pregnant or lactating woman.

    b. Cyclic antidepressants.

    c. An SSRI.

    d. MAO inhibitors.

9. The drug-receptor hypothesis is the (page 798)

    a. theory that some people are more receptive to drug effects than others.

    b. theory that drugs bind at the molecular level to receptor sites in the human body.

    c. fact that drugs can be given in a variety of routes, such as orally, by injection, or intravenously.

    d. belief that drugs will be abused unless regulated by the FDA.

10. Stimulants can be effective and prudent medications for all of the following conditions except (page 797)

    a. depression.

    b. narcolepsy.

    c. fatigue.

    d. adult Attention-Deficit Disorder.

11. Methadone maintenance may offer all the following advantages except (pages 794-795)

    a. reducing criminal behavior associated with opioid addiction.

    b. eliminating addiction.

    c. connecting addicts with health care providers.

    d. eliminating or reducing the use of needles, reducing the risk of AIDS and other diseases associated with the use of needles.

12. Identify the following drugs as either antipsychotics (P), antidepressants (D), or antianxiety (A) medications.

_____ Risperdal

_____ Elavil

_____ Loxitane

_____ Klonopin

_____ Librium

_____ Ambien

_____ Mellaril

_____ Desyrel

_____ Prozac

_____ Thorazine

_____ BuSpar

_____ Haldol

_____ Ativan

_____ Olanzapine

Chapter 28

INDIVIDUAL PSYCHOTHERAPY

The purpose of this chapter is to help you understand the effectiveness of individual psychotherapy as a treatment for psychiatric disorders. In this chapter, you will learn which disorders are effectively treated with this modality, as well as the techniques associated with individual psychotherapy. The various modes and methods of individual therapy are discussed, and the unique role of nurses in providing individual therapy is presented.

READING ASSIGNMENT

Please read Chapter 28, "Individual Psychotherapy," pages 804–818.

KEY TERMS

Write definitions for the following terms in your own words. Compare your definitions with those given in the text.

Behaviorally Oriented Therapy _____

_____

Catharsis _____

_____

Clarification _____

_____

Client-Centered Therapy _____

_____

Cognitive-Behavioral Therapy _____

_____

Confrontation _____

_____

Experience-Oriented Therapy _____

_____

Insight-Oriented Therapy _____

_____

Interpersonal Therapy _____

_____

Interpretation _____

_____

Psychoanalysis _____

_____

Psychodynamic Therapy _____

_____

Psychotherapy _____

_____

Repression _____

_____

Suggestion _____

_____

EXERCISES AND ACTIVITIES

1. The difference between psychotherapy and counseling can be vague. What is the difference as you understand it? (pages 806–807)

_____

_____

_____

_____

_____

2. Which health professionals are licensed to perform psychotherapy? (pages 806–807)

_____

_____

_____

_____

_____

   a. What qualifications does a therapist have to have?

_____

_____

_____

_____

_____

   b. What kinds of psychotherapy and/or counseling is a nurse entitled to provide, and what qualifications must the nurse have? Be sure to consider your state's Nurse Practice Act.

_____

_____

_____

_____

_____

3. Think about Salvador Dali's painting on page 807.
   a. Why do you think Dali called it *The Persistence of Memory*?

_____

_____

_____

_____

_____

b. What is it about psychoanalysis that led the authors to offer this painting as a pictorial analogy to psychotherapy?

_____

_____

_____

_____

_____

4. List the pros and cons of intensive psychoanalysis, as you see them. (pages 807–809)

a. Pros

_____

_____

_____

_____

_____

b. Cons

_____

_____

_____

_____

_____

5. Compare and contrast Freudian psychoanalytic therapy with Rogerian client-centered therapy. (page 811)

_____

_____

_____

_____

_____

6. Identify nursing theories that are consistent with the role of the nurse as individual therapist and provide a brief rationale. (page 814)

_____

_____

_____

_____

_____

7. In a collaborative psychiatric setting, who are the other mental health professionals on the team? (page 815)

_____

_____

_____

_____

_____

a. What are their roles and responsibilities?

_____

_____

_____

_____

_____

b. Which of these roles and responsibilities could be assumed by a nurse in advanced practice?

_____

_____

_____

_____

_____

c. What are the unique roles and responsibilities of the nurse on the team?

_____

_____

_____

_____

_____

8. List the disorders that evidence shows are most responsive to individual psychotherapy. (pages 807–811)

_____

_____

_____

_____

_____

9. Cite evidence supporting the efficacy of cognitive-behavioral therapy. (pages 810–811)

_____

_____

_____

_____

_____

10. State your view of the future of individual psychotherapy.

_____

_____

_____

_____

_____

SELF-ASSESSMENT QUIZ

1. A major medical textbook presents the view that the role of the therapist must be that of (page 807)

    a. advocate.

    b. curer.

    c. helper.

    d. parent.

2. During an individual session with a client, the nurse states, "You want to stop smoking but you just called your family and asked them to bring you two cartons of cigarettes." Which therapeutic communication technique is the nurse using? (page 808)

    a. Reflection

    b. Informing

    c. Focusing

    d. Confrontation

3. If a nurse states to a client, "You are angry with me because I'm telling you the same thing your mother told you," the nurse is using which technique? (page 808)

    a. Interpretation

    b. Clarification

    c. Confrontation

    d. Suggestion

4. Nursing research studies evaluating the effects of interpersonal therapy have suggested that this approach is useful for clients with (page 810)

    a. personality disorders and schizophrenia.

    b. substance abuse disorders and eating disorders.

    c. mood disorders and eating disorders.

    d. sleep disorders and sexual disorders.

5. One of the most effective therapies used with children is (page 813)

    a. reality therapy.

    b. play therapy.

    c. primal therapy.

    d. persuasion therapy.

6. Besides intensive psychotherapy, people today can choose from a variety of approaches to therapy, organized according to all of the following categories except (pages 807–811)

    a. experience-oriented therapies.

    b. denial-oriented therapies.

    c. insight-oriented therapies.

    d. task-oriented therapies.

7. Characteristics of cognitive-behavioral therapy include all of the following except (page 810)

    a. understanding the origins of current problems.

    b. short-term duration.

    c. orientation toward self-help.

    d. orientation toward practical results.

8. Of the following, which statement is *not* true regarding interpersonal therapy? (pages 809–810)

    a. Client mental health problems arise in the course of human relationships rather than in individual psychodevelopment.

    b. The therapy is based on the ideas of Sullivan, not Freud.

    c. Nurses can substitute for poor relationships elsewhere in the client's life.

    d. Nurses can model positive relationships using Peplau's theory.

9. All of the following are techniques of psychoanalysis except (page 808)

    a. coercion.

    b. confrontation.

    c. manipulation.

    d. suggestion.

10. Cognitive-behavioral therapy can be used effectively with all of the following psychiatric disorders except (page 810)

    a. substance abuse.

    b. eating disorders.

    c. psychotic thought patterns.

    d. sexual dysfunction.

Chapter 29

FAMILY THERAPY

The purpose of this chapter is to explore the role of families in psychiatric mental health nursing. Individuals with mental health problems can both affect and be affected by their families. Nurses need to understand family development and dynamics and to develop skills associated with assessing and intervening with families to promote health, prevent illness, and treat problems.

READING ASSIGNMENT

Please read Chapter 29, "Family Therapy," pages 820–851.

KEY TERMS

Write definitions for the following terms in your own words. Compare your definitions with those given in the text.

Circular Communication _____

_____

Differentiation _____

_____

Ecomap _____

_____

Emotional Cutoff _____

_____

Family _____

_____

Family Attachment Diagram _____

_____

Family Projection Process _____

_____

Genogram _____

_____

Interventive Questions _____

_____

Multigenerational Transmission Process _____

_____

Nuclear Family Emotional System _____

_____

Power _____

_____

Relativistic Thinking _____

_____

Sibling Position_____

_____

Societal Regression _____

_____

Triangulation _____

_____

EXERCISES AND ACTIVITIES

1. The definition of *family* is very broad. (page 822)

   a. For the purposes of providing effective nursing care, why must this be so?

   _____

   _____

   _____

   _____

   _____

b. In cases where family membership is ambiguous, how can the nurse determine who are family members?

_____

_____

_____

_____

_____

c. Do you hold any value judgments about what a family is that you think could interfere with your ability to provide care to a family group? What decisions can you make right now that would enable you to provide professional nursing care if a client's family values clashed with your own?

_____

_____

_____

_____

_____

2. Review Table 29-1, "Four Approaches to Family Nursing in Psychiatric Mental Health Care," on page 825. Cover the middle column and define each approach's use in psychiatric nursing in your own words. Check yourself with the information given in the table.

3. Using your family or a family close to you as an example, answer the following questions about family development: (pages 825–826)

a. What stage of family development is your family in?

_____

_____

_____

_____

_____

b. What tasks must your family master before moving on to the next stage?

_____

_____

_____

_____

_____

c. In what ways, if any, would Duvall's Family Development Theory be inadequate to sufficiently account for current developmental issues in your family? (pages 825–826)

_____

_____

_____

_____

_____

4. Study Table 29-3, "Level of Differentiation and Family Patterns," on page 829.

a. Explain the general differences among families in terms of low, moderate, and high levels of differentiation.

_____

_____

_____

_____

_____

b. What application does the concept of differentiation have to caring for families?

_____

_____

_____

_____

_____

5. Using the figures presented on page 834, draw a genogram of your family, carrying it out to three generations.

6. Using your family genogram, make a family attachment diagram, using yourself as the focal point. (page 834)

7. Explain the relationship between family assessment and family intervention. (pages 833–841)

_____

_____

_____

_____

_____

8. Draw an ecomap with your family in the middle. (page 835)

a. What surprised you about your family's ecomap?

_____

_____

_____

_____

_____

b. What changes would you like to make, if any, in the strength of connections between various elements in your family's ecomap? (page 836)

_____

_____

_____

_____

_____

9. Think about the trifocal model in terms of your family. (page 836)

a. What are the wellness patterns in your family?

_____

_____

_____

_____

_____

b. What areas of prevention do you think your family would benefit from?

_____

_____

_____

_____

_____

c. What family problems can you identify in your family?

_____

_____

_____

_____

_____

10. List NANDA nursing diagnoses that, although originally developed to be applied to individuals, might also be used with family units. (pages 835–837)

_____

_____

_____

_____

_____

SELF-ASSESSMENT QUIZ

1. A woman whose divorce was finalized a week ago arrives at the clinic and states to the nurse, "I've just had a very messy divorce. I have custody of our children and I was awarded the house and furniture. Is it possible to get a prescription because my nerves are shattered?" The nurse recognizes that according to Bowen's Theory of Family Development, the woman must address which of the following tasks in order to successfully continue her life? (page 827)

    a. Mourn the loss of the nuclear family

    b. Rebuild her own social network

    c. Renegotiate the marital system as a dyad

    d. Accept her part in the failure of the marriage

2. An appropriate nursing outcome for a reconstituted family would be which of the following? (page 828)

    a. The family will be able to restructure family boundaries to allow for inclusion of the new spouse and stepparent.

    b. The family will learn to forget their previous family structure and replace it with the new structure.

    c. Family members will acknowledge the superiority of the reconstituted family compared to the original family structure.

    d. Family members will learn to live more independently from their newly reconstituted family.

3. During a family therapy session, the husband states, "Every time we argue, my wife has to run to her mother. I'm tired of my mother-in-law always sticking her nose in our business." The nurse therapist would hypothesize that the wife's behavior of involving her mother is an example of which of the following according to Bowen? (page 828)

   a. Disenfranchisement

   b. Differentiation

   c. Triangulation

   d. Emotional cutoff

4. Which nursing approach would the nurse initiate when caring for a family at a low level of differentiation? (page 826)

   a. Facilitate family members' own abilities to feel emotions and understand events.

   b. Seek to develop trust with the family and provide experiences that will help the adults develop cognitive skills to understand their emotions.

   c. Condition family members to become less reliant on the family structure and family members in providing their needs.

   d. Identify and isolate family members that are behaving in manners counterproductive to family well-being.

5. The nurse caring for families at a high level of differentiation would recognize that these families (page 829)

   a. live in the present and do not think ahead.

   b. demonstrate realistic thinking.

   c. exhibit family dynamics that are impulsive.

   d. exhibit family dynamics that are rigid.

6. A modern definition of family would exclude which of the following individuals from membership in the family? (page 822)

   a. People not related by blood

   b. People not living together

   c. Disinherited children

   d. People who the family members agree are not part of the family

7. Families with a low level of differentiation are characterized by (page 826)

   a. acting like 2-year-olds.

   b. acting impulsively, emotionally, and selfishly.

   c. lack of ability to function in all aspects of life.

   d. intense but short-term relationships.

8. The following are among Bowen's concepts of familial and emotional interaction patterns except (page 826)

   a. strangulation.

   b. triangulation.

   c. emotional cutoff.

   d. differentiation.

9. Nurses can positively affect families in all of the following ways except which? (pages 829–830)

   a. Nurses can help identify family strengths.

   b. Nurses can identify and point out patterns and rules within families that may be unhealthy but are unseen by the family itself.

   c. Nurses can become a surrogate member of the family.

   d. Nurses can identify the source of individual problems within the context of family problems.

10. All of the following family perspectives are useful to the nurse except (pages 823–824)

    a. family as a component of society.

    b. family as a political group.

    c. family as context.

    d. family as client.

Chapter 30

GROUP THERAPY

The purpose of this chapter is to explain how groups can accomplish therapeutic purposes and to show nurses the techniques and approaches to group work that can help facilitate positive outcomes.

READING ASSIGNMENT

Please read Chapter 30, "Group Therapy," pages 852–868.

KEY TERMS

Write definitions for the following terms in your own words. Compare your definitions with those given in the text.

Closed Group _____

_____

Group _____

_____

Group Content _____

_____

Group Dynamics _____

_____

Group Leader/Facilitator _____

_____

Group Process _____

_____

Open Group _____

_____

Self-Help Group _____

_____

Supportive Group _____

_____

Therapy Group_____

_____

EXERCISES AND ACTIVITIES

1. Name as many different kinds of client groups as you can think of. (page 852)

    _____

    _____

    _____

    _____

    _____

2. Review Table 30-1, "Three Phases of Group Work," on page 855. Compare these stages with Peplau's interpersonal relations in nursing stages on pages 30–31.

    _____

    _____

    _____

    _____

    _____

3. In your own words, state the "roles" that help facilitate the group process. (pages 856–857)

    _____

    _____

    _____

    _____

    _____

4. An effective technique that nurses can use to facilitate groups is to comment on the group process. Compose a facilitating statement to respond to the following situations. (pages 856–857)

   a. The group has gotten off-track.

   _____

   _____

   b. The group has fallen silent.

   _____

   _____

   c. Two members of the group are arguing.

   _____

   _____

   d. One member of the group is dominating.

   _____

   _____

   e. One member of the group is not participating verbally but is making many nonverbal and body language gestures.

   _____

   _____

   f. One member of the group is not participating verbally or nonverbally.

   _____

   _____

   g. All the group members seem to be hostile toward or unsupportive of one group member.

   _____

   _____

h. One group member is hostile toward or argumentative with all other group members.

_____

_____

5. You may be familiar with television shows that depict group therapy. Even though the shows are intended to be funny or dramatic, the group therapy is intended to mimic real therapy approaches. To the best of your ability, identify the group therapy approaches used in the following shows, explaining the rationale for your answer.

   a. *Frasier* (radio show, "I'm listening ... ")

   _____

   _____

   _____

   _____

   _____

   b. *The Bob Newhart Show* (psychologist conducts group therapy in his office)

   _____

   _____

   _____

   _____

   _____

   c. *Dr. Phil*

   _____

   _____

   _____

   _____

   _____

6. A self-help group is formed for people seeking support and solutions from peers facing similar problems. List client problems you have seen in your clinical experience that you think might benefit from the formation of a self-help group. (page 862)

---

7. Give examples of "socialization" groups you or your parents or significant others may have arranged for you when you were growing up whose purpose it was to help you approach some developmental task. (page 861)

---

8. What kind(s) of group would an Outward Bound or wilderness survival experience be? (page 862)

---

9. What is the purpose of silence in a group?

---

10. Explain the difference between group process and group dynamics. (page 856)

_____

_____

_____

_____

_____

SELF-ASSESSMENT QUIZ

1. During a group session, a client is told by another group member that the client needs to change his behavior. Hearing this, the client becomes tearful and begins to cry. The nurse interprets the client's behavior as which of the following?

    a. The client feels too fragile to be challenged.

    b. The client's feelings have been hurt by the other group member.

    c. The client feels extreme depression regarding his own behavior.

    d. The client is angry that he has been confronted by another group member.

2. A new nurse graduate is planning to run a small group meeting with several clients on the unit. The nurse understands that the goal for this type of treatment is which of the following? (page 858)

    a. Developing insight

    b. Providing clients with professional advice

    c. Maintaining control over group members' comments

    d. Providing an opportunity to develop friendships

3. The technique of psychodrama originated with the work of (page 860)

    a. Peplau.

    b. Freud.

    c. Moreno.

    d. Sullivan.

4. The emphasis of psychodrama is on (page 860)

   a. family relationships.

   b. the here and now.

   c. past traumatic experiences

   d. dream interpretation.

5. During which phase of the group process do group members acknowledge the contributions of each member? (page 856)

   a. Pre-orientation

   b. Orientation

   c. Working

   d. Termination

6. All of the following are valid approaches to therapy groups except (pages 858–860)

   a. existential groups.

   b. interpersonal groups.

   c. psychodrama.

   d. confessional approach.

7. Which of the following is an effective group therapy for elderly patients because it focuses on the here and now? (page 862)

   a. Trauma therapy

   b. Gestalt therapy

   c. Movement therapy

   d. Game therapy

8. The reasons that psychoanalytic therapy can work well in a group include all of the following except which? (pages 858–859)

   a. Clients may be unwilling to disclose embarrassing personal information in a group setting.

   b. Clients may feel empowered to disclose embarrassing personal information if they see that someone else was able to do so and be supported.

   c. Clients may receive more varied and helpful feedback to their disclosures.

   d. Clients may come to understand that they are not alone in their feelings.

9. Psychodrama is an effective group modality for many clients for all these reasons except which? (page 860)

   a. It is impossible for the client to hide from past disturbing events by erecting a barrier to years of feelings, denials, and repression.

   b. Reliving past uncomfortable events is accomplished in a safe, supportive setting.

   c. It offers clients an opportunity to change or alter past traumatic experiences.

   d. It offers clients an opportunity to achieve closure to past traumatic experiences.

10. The group leader who reaches the termination phase of a group should do all of the following except (page 856)

   a. plan for the group's termination, perhaps by organizing a ceremony or small party.

   b. recognize that feelings of change, sadness, and anxiety may accompany the termination of a group.

   c. suggest or plan a group reunion at a future date so that it does not really feel as if the group is terminating.

   d. ask members to state the ways they may have benefited from being part of the group.

Chapter 31

COMMUNITY MENTAL HEALTH NURSING

The purpose of this chapter is to help you understand how the concept of community health nursing can be applied to psychiatric mental health nursing. Community psychiatric mental health nursing is of particular importance following the massive deinstitutionalization in the 1970s of people severely ill with mental illness, shifting the need for psychiatric nursing resources from hospitals to the community.

READING ASSIGNMENT

Please read Chapter 31, "Community Mental Health Nursing," pages 870–885.

KEY TERMS

Write definitions for the following terms in your own words. Compare your definitions with those given in the text.

Aggregate _____

_____

Assertive Community Treatment (ACT) _____

_____

Capitation _____

_____

Case Management _____

_____

Community Health Nursing _____

_____

Community Mental Health _____

_____

Community Support System (CSS) _____

_____

Deinstitutionalization _____

_____

Home Health Nursing _____

_____

Managed Care_____

_____

Population _____

_____

Primary Prevention _____

_____

Program for Assertive Community Treatment (PACT) _____

_____

Prospective Payment System _____

_____

Public Health Nursing _____

_____

Secondary Prevention _____

_____

Tertiary Prevention _____

_____

EXERCISES AND ACTIVITIES

1. What resources exist in your community to care for people with mental illnesses?

    _____

    _____

    _____

    _____

    _____

2. List the common barriers you see that mentally ill people have to overcome to access mental health services in their communities. (pages 874–876)

_____

_____

_____

_____

_____

3. List important legislation that led to the creation of mental health resources in the community to your timeline. (pages 873–875)

_____

_____

_____

_____

_____

4. What kind of nursing support is needed by individuals with schizophrenia who function adequately when taking their medication? (pages 874–875)

_____

_____

_____

_____

_____

5. Define *case management*. (page 876)

_____

_____

_____

_____

_____

a. List the six areas of responsibility for case managers.

_____

_____

_____

_____

_____

6. Compare and contrast a community support system (CSS) with a Program for Assertive Community Treatment (PACT). (pages 875–876)

_____

_____

_____

_____

_____

7. What are the rights of people with mental illnesses? (page 879)

_____

_____

_____

_____

_____

8. President George W. Bush established the New Freedom Commission on Mental Health in 2002.

a. What national mental health problems did the commission identify?

_____

_____

_____

_____

_____

b. What recommendations did the commission make?

_____

_____

_____

_____

_____

c. Which of these recommendations have been implemented in your community?

_____

_____

_____

_____

_____

9. List the stressors experienced by family members caring for relatives with mental illnesses. (page 880)

_____

_____

_____

_____

_____

a. How should community mental health agencies address the needs of caregivers?

_____

_____

_____

_____

_____

b. What can nurses do to ease the burden of caregivers?

_____

_____

_____

_____

_____

10. What responsibilities, roles, and tasks are associated with the position of psychiatric home care provider?

_____

_____

_____

_____

_____

SELF-ASSESSMENT QUIZ

1. A community nurse working as a mental health case manager would include which of the following activities as part of the nurse's advocacy role? (page 876)

    a. Calling the client who missed an appointment to determine why the appointment was missed

    b. Speaking to a client's landlord to arrange for necessary repairs for the client's apartment

    c. Making an appointment for a client with a vocational rehabilitation counselor

    d. Holding a care conference for a client who is having difficulty adjusting to a new job situation

2. When a hospital or health care facility receives funds to provide specific services for a specific population, this source of funding is known as which of the following? (page 880)

    a. Capitation funding

    b. Managed care funding

    c. Fee-for-service funding

    d. Prospective payment funding

3. Which of the following resulted in the creation of community support systems (CSSs)? (page 874)

    a. A shortage of physicians and nurses resulting from a decrease in federal funding for training of health professions

    b. Inadequate resources following massive deinstitutionalization in the late 1960s and 1970s

    c. Increased immigration of individuals from Mexico and Cuba in the 1980s

    d. Changes in the structure of families due to increases in the divorce and adoption rates in the 1970s and 1980s

4. Public health services that focus on a rehabilitative approach to daily living include which of the following? (page 780)

    a. Educating about medication

    b. Reducing residual defects associated with mental disorder

    c. Providing crisis management

    d. Developing relations with landlords

5. For nurses to function effectively as interdisciplinary team members, they will need to (page 882)

    a. keep their traditional role as care providers.

    b. become leaders of all interdisciplinary groups.

    c. overcome personality and turf barriers.

    d. return to school to obtain a doctorate.

6. The founder of modern public health or community health nursing is (page 872)

    a. Florence Nightingale.

    b. Hildegard Peplau.

    c. Lillian Wald.

    d. Margaret Sanger.

7. Many social forces work against successful care of the mentally ill population in the community. These forces include all of the following except (pages 872–875)

    a. unqualified or unwilling caregivers in the clients' families.

    b. discrimination against people with mental illness.

    c. health insurance company practices.

    d. mental health advocacy groups.

8. Which of the following in *not* a mission of the National Alliance for the Mentally Ill (NAMI)? (page 877)

    a. establishing civil rights for people with mental illness.

    b. promoting deinstitutionalization.

    c. fighting against the stigmatization of the mentally ill.

    d. lobbying governments for more effective legislation for the treatment of people with psychiatric disorders.

9. All of the following statements about the public health model are true except which? (pages 880–881)

    a. The community, not the individual, is the focus of treatment.

    b. The model does not apply to populations of people who are already severely mentally ill.

    c. The emphasis of the model is on prevention.

    d. The concept of prevention can apply to people who are already severely mentally ill.

10. In the twenty-first century, psychiatric nurses working in the community will face all of the following challenges except which? (page 882)

    a. Care will be increasingly collaborative.

    b. Nurses working with the mentally ill in the community will be paid better than social workers, psychologists, and nurses working in hospitals.

    c. Nurses will focus more on rehabilitative services.

    d. Nurses will work more often for managed-care firms.

Chapter 32

COMPLEMENTARY AND SOMATIC THERAPIES

The purpose of this chapter is to familiarize the nurse with the somatic therapies long used in psychiatric care and the generally newer complementary therapies used mainly by nurses to add to the diversity of medical and psychiatric therapies. These interventions and treatments augment conventional psychiatric practice and nursing and broaden the scope of psychiatric nursing. All of the complementary therapies are classified as nursing interventions by NIC and have been shown to be effective in treating specific psychiatric disorders and symptoms.

READING ASSIGNMENT

Please read Chapter 32, "Complementary and Somatic Therapies," pages 886–904.

KEY TERMS

Write definitions for the following terms in your own words. Compare your definitions with those given in the text.

Anger Control Assistance _____

_____

Animal-Assisted Therapy _____

_____

Complementary Modalities_____

_____

Electroconvulsive Therapy (ECT) _____

_____

Energy-Based Modalities _____

_____

Guided Imagery _____

_____

Healing Touch_____

_____

Hypnosis_____

_____

Light Therapy (Phototherapy) _____

_____

Massage _____

_____

Music Therapy _____

_____

Relaxation _____

_____

Seclusion_____

_____

Somatic Therapies _____

_____

Therapeutic Imagery_____

_____

Therapeutic Massage_____

_____

Therapeutic Touch (TT) _____

_____

EXERCISES AND ACTIVITIES

1. When you feel overwhelmed with stress, how do you treat yourself? What relaxes you? (pages 886–896)

   _____

   _____

   _____

   _____

   _____

2. What characteristics of Frederick Varley's painting *Dhârâna*, on page 890, suggest relaxation?

   _____

   _____

   _____

   _____

   _____

3. Read the material on guided imagery on pages 890–891.

   a. What are the differences between guided imagery and relaxation therapy?

   _____

   _____

   _____

   _____

   _____

b. What is the pleasant "place" in your mind that you would visit if you were practicing guided imagery on yourself?

_____

_____

_____

_____

_____

_____

c. What techniques can be used to enhance the effectiveness of guided imagery?

_____

_____

_____

_____

_____

_____

d. What are some characteristics of people who can image responsively?

_____

_____

_____

_____

_____

_____

4. What are your state's licensing, educational, and supervisory requirements to practice hypnosis or hypnotherapy?

_____

_____

_____

_____

_____

5. What is the difference between massage and therapeutic massage? (pages 892–893)

_____

_____

_____

_____

_____

a. What training have you received in massage as a nursing student?

_____

_____

_____

_____

_____

b. What conditions can be treated effectively with therapeutic massage?

_____

_____

_____

_____

_____

6. The authors state, "Simple touch—reaching out to physically contact another—is a therapy too often neglected in busy nursing practice." Do you agree? Why or why not? (page 892)

_____

_____

_____

_____

_____

7. Have you ever used music therapy to treat a sleep disturbance you have experienced? If so, what aspects of your self-treatment did you find effective? (page 895)

_____

_____

_____

_____

_____

8. What signals are there that a client is at risk for becoming violent? (page 896)

_____

_____

_____

_____

_____

9. Review the material on physical restraints on page 897.

   a. What requirement must be satisfied before physical restraints can be used?

   _____

   _____

   _____

   _____

   _____

   b. What techniques are associated with the therapeutic or safe and professional use of restraints on clients?

   _____

   _____

   _____

   _____

   _____

c. What message should be directed toward a client who is being restrained?

_____

_____

_____

_____

_____

d. What conditions and practices must be observed while a client is in restraints?

_____

_____

_____

_____

_____

10. When is electroconvulsive therapy (ECT) indicated? (pages 898–899)

_____

_____

_____

_____

_____

a. What is your personal opinion of ECT?

_____

_____

_____

_____

_____

b. What are the risks of ECT?

_____

_____

_____

_____

_____

c. Considering how painful mental illness can be, has your opinion of ECT changed since you began this course but before you read this chapter? If so, in what ways?

_____

_____

_____

_____

_____

SELF-ASSESSMENT QUIZ

1. Which individual developed the technique of therapeutic touch (TT)? (page 894)

    a. Martha Rogers

    b. Dolores Krieger

    c. Dora Kung

    d. Janet Quinn

2. The best music to achieve a relaxation response in music therapy has (page 895)

    a. a strong rhythm with beats that are slower than the heart rate.

    b. a strong rhythm with beats that are faster than the heart rate.

    c. a weak rhythm with beats that are slower than the heart rate.

    d. a moderate rhythm with beats that are identical to the heart rate.

3. Progressive muscle relaxation (PMR) has been effective in treating clients who are (page 889)

    a. anxious.

    b. depressed.

    c. incontinent.

    d. sleep deprived.

4. Reed's 2007 study "Imagery in the Clinical Setting: A Tool for Healing" found that (page 891)

    a. there were no changes in the habits of either the experimental or control group.

    b. the control group demonstrated a significant decrease in perception and an increase in daily use of opioid pain medication post surgery.

    c. the experimental group demonstrated a significant decrease in perception and a decrease in daily use of opioid pain medication post surgery.

    d. both groups experienced an increased need for pain medication post surgery.

5. Findings from Kay's 2007 study "Effectiveness of Hypnosis in Reducing Mild Essential Hypertension: A One-Year Follow-Up Study" revealed that (page 892)

    a. for the experimental subjects, both systolic and diastolic pressure increased after the hypnosis treatment.

    b. for the experimental subjects, both systolic and diastolic pressure were reduced after the hypnosis treatment.

    c. for the control subjects, systolic and diastolic pressure remained the same as those of the experimental subjects.

    d. for the experimental subjects, systolic pressure increased and diastolic pressure decreased after the hypnosis treatment.

6. Of the following, which physiological change does *not* take place during relaxation therapy? (pages 888–890)

    a. One becomes aware that one has been tense or stressed.

    b. The parasympathetic nervous system gains dominance over the sympathetic nervous system.

    c. Blood pressure, heart rate, and respiratory rate decrease.

    d. Alpha waves in the brain increase.

7. Guided imagery should never be used with people who are (page 891)

    a. going through labor and childbirth.

    b. experiencing psychotic thought processes.

    c. experiencing pain.

    d. depressed.

8. Music therapy is used for (page 895)

    a. entertainment.

    b. diversion.

    c. a measurable relaxation response.

    d. reducing anxiety in the operating room.

9. All of the following are true of electroconvulsive therapy (ECT) except which? (pages 898–899)

    a. Nobody knows why it works.

    b. It seems most effective in clients with depression and bipolar illness.

    c. It should be used to punish incorrigible clients because it works by means of a guilt mechanism.

    d. A controlled seizure seems to produce the therapeutic effect.

10. Post-ECT nursing care includes all of the following except (page 899)

    a. monitoring brain activity with electroencephalograms.

    b. orienting client to time, place, and person.

    c. monitoring vital signs.

    d. monitoring behavior, including confusion, until short-term memory returns to normal.

Chapter 33

FRIDAY NIGHT AT THE MOVIES

The purpose of this chapter is to explore the concepts of psychiatric mental health nursing through over 100 films that present specific conditions, disorders, symptoms, and responses to mental health and illness. This review shows that mental stressors are not the exclusive property of the mentally ill—we all experience mental stressors, and the level of our mental health, as these movies show, determines our ability to cope with them. Moreover, taken together, the films form a general review of this textbook.

READING ASSIGNMENT

Please read Chapter 33, "Friday Night at the Movies," pages 906-930.

KEY TERMS

Don't forget to use the textbook's comprehensive Glossary on pages 964-976. Frequently using this tool will help you gain a professional working knowledge of the language of psychiatry and psychiatric nursing.

EXERCISES AND ACTIVITIES

1. Why do you think the authors chose Friday night for you to spend at the movies?

   _____

   _____

   _____

   _____

   _____

2. Go to the movies with a friend or colleague to see a film that has a theme related to psychiatric mental health. Discuss the movie with your friend, based on your new knowledge of the concepts of this course. How did your reaction differ from that of your friend or colleague?

_____

_____

_____

_____

_____

3. Rent a movie that will offer insight into an area of the course you find particularly puzzling or difficult. Which movie did you choose and why?

_____

_____

_____

_____

_____

COMPREHENSIVE NCLEX STYLE PRACTICE FINAL EXAMINATION

1. An instructor is evaluating whether the nursing students understand neurotransmitters. The instructor would recognize that learning has occurred if the students answered that neurotransmitters are

    1. electrical signals in the brain.

    2. chemical messengers in the brain.

    3. neurons.

    4. synapses.

2. When asked what is the current version of the American Psychiatric Association's Diagnostic Statistical Manual, a student nurse is correct if he or she answers

    1. DSM-IIIR.

    2. DSM-IV.

    3. DSM-IV-TR.

    4. DSM-V.

3. A student nurse asks the charge nurse what is involved with Axis IV of the DSM. The charge nurse would most likely reply that it identifies

    1. general psychiatric disorders.

    2. general medical disorders.

    3. psychosocial and environmental problems.

    4. global problems.

4. A surprising fact about NANDA's nursing diagnoses is

   1. even though they are designed for use with clients who have any kind of health problem, over half of them pertain to psychosocial issues.

   2. someday the NANDA diagnoses will replace the DSM-IV-TR.

   3. the NANDA diagnoses exclude human responses to mental disorders.

   4. the NANDA diagnoses will expire in the year 2015.

5. A nursing student's assessment of a client reveals that the client is utilizing several defense mechanisms. The nursing student would recognize that defense mechanisms

   1. refer to the immune system's ability to ward off disease.

   2. are inborn.

   3. protect people from mental illnesses.

   4. unconsciously protect people from internal conflicts and external stressors.

6. The Carter Commission

   1. identified the "tip-of-the-iceberg" phenomenon.

   2. promoted deinstitutionalization.

   3. identified the prevalence and incidence of mental illnesses.

   4. made psychiatric nursing part of the general nursing curriculum.

7. A nursing instructor would include in the teaching plan for the course that under all but the most dire circumstances, clients have the right to

   1. disrupt the treatment programs of other clients.

   2. smoke.

   3. refuse treatment.

   4. be judged by a panel of their peers.

8. To control violent or self-destructive behavior in clients, nurses are obligated to use

   1. the least restrictive alternative.

   2. any means necessary.

   3. their best judgment.

   4. the physician's written order.

9. Hans Selye's General Adaptation Syndrome is
    1. a medical diagnosis.
    2. a psychiatric diagnosis.
    3. a model of a healthy response to stress.
    4. irrelevant in some cultures.

10. The key difference between anxiety and fear is that
    1. fear is normal, anxiety is not.
    2. fear is more often experienced by males, whereas anxiety is more often experienced by females.
    3. fear involves dread of some specific threat, whereas anxiety occurs without relation to a specific threat.
    4. fear is a nursing diagnosis, whereas anxiety is a medical diagnosis.

11. An appropriate intervention for someone seeking emergency care for acute stress would be
    1. to assure the client that the future will be better.
    2. to help the client cognitively reframe the stressful situation.
    3. sedation.
    4. meditation.

12. A client is admitted to the psychiatric unit with a diagnosis of Panic Disorder. The nurse recognizes that this disorder is
    1. anxiety accompanied by crying.
    2. unrelated to anxiety.
    3. a form of anxiety characterized by intense episodes and specific physiological symptoms.
    4. anxiety accompanied by psychosis.

13. It is appropriate to diagnose Obsessive-Compulsive Disorder when
    1. fear of self-contamination is consistent with risk.
    2. clients can't remember whether they turned off the oven.
    3. clients go through rituals.
    4. fear of self-contamination is inconsistent with risk.

14. When planning care for a client with anxiety, the nurse recognizes that treatment for this disorder depends on
    1. the client's tolerance of drugs.
    2. whether the client uses alcohol or not.
    3. the client's specific diagnosis.
    4. the severity of the anxiety.

15. A client approaches a nurse and states, "Coming time fizzle dock helper." The nurse assesses the client's speech as
    1. neologizing.
    2. word salad.
    3. tangentiality.
    4. derailment.

16. When assessing a client, the nurse would most likely identify which of the following as a "positive" symptom of schizophrenia?
    1. Hallucinations
    2. Flat affect
    3. Lack of relationships
    4. Withdrawal

17. A nurse would assess which of the following as a "negative" symptom of schizophrenia?
    1. Disordered thought
    2. Delusions
    3. Anhedonia
    4. Bizarre behavior

18. A nurse caring for a schizophrenic client recognizes that the dopamine hypothesis for schizophrenia suggests that
    1. schizophrenia strikes at random.
    2. dopamine production is higher in the brains of people with schizophrenia.
    3. dopamine production is lower in the brains of people with schizophrenia.
    4. dopamine apparently has nothing to do with schizophrenia.

19. When administering medications to clients, the nurse recognizes that which of the following is *not* true of neuroleptic medications?

    1. Generally, most are more effective against the positive rather than the negative symptoms of schizophrenia.

    2. Their mechanism often causes severe neuromuscular side effects.

    3. They are the only treatment for schizophrenia that has proven effective.

    4. They work by blocking dopamine, a neurotransmitter, at the brain's dopamine receptors.

20. When a nurse has diagnosed a client with altered thought processes, the nurse should respond to the client by

    1. redirecting the client's attention back to the here and now.

    2. exploring the client's delusions with him or her.

    3. arguing with the client about his or her disordered thoughts.

    4. speaking louder to be heard above the voices the client is hearing.

21. When planning care for clients in the rehabilitative phase of schizophrenia, the nurse should

    1. allow the clients to spend time alone in a private space.

    2. give the clients responsibility for getting to their appointments on time.

    3. help the clients structure their day with a written schedule.

    4. befriend the client.

22. An instructor evaluates that a student understands the difference between unipolar depression and bipolar depression if the student responds that

    1. in unipolar depression, the client is always hypomanic.

    2. in unipolar depression, the client swings from one end of the mood continuum to the other.

    3. in bipolar depression, the client has upswings, or highs, at least some of the time.

    4. in bipolar depression, the client swings between depression and anxiety.

23. The nurse assessing a client with Major Depressive Disorder recognizes that the symptoms can include
    1. hunger.
    2. thought disorder.
    3. suicidal thoughts.
    4. grandiosity.

24. When teaching a client's family the differences between Major Depressive Disorder and Dysthymic Disorder, the nurse would include the fact that
    1. Dysthymic Disorder is just a short episode of depression.
    2. Dysthymic Disorder is a chronic depression lasting more than two years.
    3. Dysthymic Disorder is a depression brought on by a food allergy.
    4. Dysthymic Disorder is a side effect of psychotropic medications.

25. In preparing client teaching about the concept of grief, the nurse would teach that the stages of grief include all of the following except
    1. recovery.
    2. reality.
    3. chronic.
    4. shock.

26. Freud conceived the superego to be
    1. the conscience.
    2. conceit.
    3. the supreme being.
    4. the cerebral cortex.

27. A client is admitted with a diagnosis of depression. Which group of medications would be least likely to be part of the treatment plan?
    1. MAO inhibitors
    2. Phenothiazines
    3. Tricyclics
    4. Selective serotonin reuptake inhibitors

28. For planning the nursing care of clients with depression, nurses may find it useful to think in terms of Orem's Self-Care Deficit Theory because

    1. depressed clients usually can't take care of themselves.

    2. nurses need to take over the care of clients with depression.

    3. clients with depression need to be expected to take care of themselves.

    4. the self-care of clients with depression needs to be thoughtfully planned.

29. A client's husband asks the nurse how mania differs from hypomania. The most accurate response by the nurse would be which of the following?

    1. The number and length of manic behaviors are fewer and shorter in hypomania.

    2. There is no difference.

    3. Unlike mania, hypomania is not a DSM-IV-TR diagnosis and is very similar to general happiness.

    4. Mania includes psychosis, whereas hypomania does not.

30. When a client transitions from mania to depression or depression to mania, the nurse assesses this as

    1. cyclothymic patterns.

    2. Bipolar Disorder.

    3. the switch process.

    4. manic-depressive illness.

31. A nurse working on a psychiatric unit recognizes that there is strong evidence suggesting that Bipolar Disorder is caused by

    1. genetic factors.

    2. environmental factors.

    3. developmental factors.

    4. learned behavior.

32. A nurse assessing clients in the emergency department understands that all of the following can produce symptoms similar to mania except

    1. drugs.

    2. physical diseases.

    3. sleep deprivation.

    4. financial difficulties.

33. A nurse teaching a community group about drugs that can cause switching from a depressive episode to a manic state would include all of the following except

    1. lithium.
    2. anabolic steroids.
    3. tricyclic antidepressants.
    4. St. John's wort.

34. When discharge teaching about Lithium, which response by the client would indicate that further teaching is needed?

    1. Lithium is ineffective in eliminating mood swings.
    2. Lithium can cloud cognitive functioning.
    3. Lithium is embryotoxic in the first trimester.
    4. Physical side effects can include hypothyroidism, kidney problems, and nervous system symptoms.

35. The nurse admits a client with Bipolar Disorder. The nurse hypothesizes that the primary treatment will include

    1. psychotherapy.
    2. electroconvulsive therapy (ECT).
    3. medications.
    4. behavioral therapy.

36. A nursing intervention effective with clients who are manic is to

    1. challenge the client's intrusive behavior and racing thoughts.
    2. use group therapy.
    3. urge the client to get more sleep.
    4. reduce unnecessary stimulation in the therapeutic environment.

37. A nurse manager preparing to teach a group of staff nurses about prevention of suicide would include which of the following as a method of tertiary prevention?

    1. Removing sharp or dangerous objects from the environment
    2. Assessing clients for suicide risk
    3. Learning CPR and other emergency medical procedures
    4. Monitoring clients closely

38. An effective intervention nurses can use to lower the risk of clients committing suicide would be

    1. keeping a watchful eye.

    2. establishing a suicide contract with clients to ensure safety for a specific period of time.

    3. hoping your relationship is strong enough with clients that they wouldn't commit suicide while you are on duty.

    4. healing touch.

39. In assessing a newly admitted client diagnosed with drug dependence, the nurse recognizes that a strong indicator of dependence on a substance or drug would be that the client

    1. has used an addictive substance.

    2. uses the substance secretively.

    3. frequents places where substances are frequently abused.

    4. tries unsuccessfully to stop using a substance.

40. A nurse working in triage would use the CAGE questionnaire to

    1. assess for claustrophobia.

    2. count words per minute for a person experiencing mania.

    3. detect alcoholism.

    4. determine the type of substance abused.

41. In teaching a client about opiate addiction, the nurse would explain that opiates are powerfully addicting substances because they

    1. fit perfectly into endorphin receptors.

    2. can be taken by many different routes of administration.

    3. are highly concentrated psychoactive substances.

    4. have been accepted in general use for many generations.

42. A nurse evaluates that a client understands Methadone maintenance if the client states that
    1. it prevents withdrawal symptoms while blocking the pleasurable effects of opiates, allowing the client to function without drug euphoria.
    2. many addicts divert methadone to the street while secretly taking opiates.
    3. it enables addicts to substitute one street drug for another.
    4. it enables addicts to practice behaviors associated with drug use.

43. The nurse preparing a teaching plan for a group of adolescents would include in the teaching plan that the principal danger of using hallucinogens is
    1. dangerous behavior due to poor judgment or faulty perceptions.
    2. addiction or dependence.
    3. they lead to the use of other drugs.
    4. never returning to normal.

44. When developing a teaching plan for a group of adolescents regarding drug abuse, the nurse would plan to include the fact that up to 50% of people who abuse drugs
    1. abuse more than one drug and/or have another psychiatric diagnosis.
    2. are women.
    3. are in prison.
    4. have a major medical disorder.

45. A family member of a client diagnosed with alcoholism asks the nurse what is meant by *codependence*. The nurse would be correct in responding that codependence is
    1. the phenomenon of being dependent on two or more drugs at one time.
    2. two people sharing a substance dependence.
    3. the relationship between a substance abuser and a significant other who facilitates the substance abuse.
    4. the relationship between a substance abuser and a spouse abuser.

46. The nurse assessing a client admitted to the unit with a diagnosis of personality disorder would hypothesize that the client's disorder first manifested itself in
    1. old age.
    2. infancy.
    3. adolescence and early adulthood.
    4. early childhood.

47. Personality disorders are classified as Axis II disorders in the DSM-IV-TR because

    1. major psychiatric disorders on Axis I are constant across all personality types.

    2. people with personality disorders don't have major psychiatric disorders like those on Axis I.

    3. Axis II disorders color Axis I disorders.

    4. a and c

48. The nurse caring for a client with Antisocial Personality Disorder recognizes that this disorder is classified as which of the following groups of personality disorders?

    1. Anxiety and fear-based group

    2. Odd and eccentric group

    3. Dramatic and emotional group

    4. None of these

49. In Borderline Personality Disorder, the term *borderline* was coined because the client is living on the border between

    1. schizophrenia and depression.

    2. anxiety and mania.

    3. psychosis and neurosis.

    4. sanity and insanity.

50. In developing a plan of care for a client with Narcissistic Personality Disorder, the nurse recognizes that people with Narcissistic Personality Disorder are probably overrepresented in the psychiatric care community because they

    1. want to be the center of attention.

    2. have difficulty forming relationships.

    3. have difficulty dealing with life stressors.

    4. are predominantly female and have fewer problems seeking help.

51. The nurse is caring for a client with Antisocial Personality Disorder. The nurse would understand that individuals with Antisocial Personality Disorder often view the nurse as

    1. a person who can help them transcend the disorder.

    2. an obstacle to being able to pursue their ends.

    3. a means to an end, like everybody else.

    4. someone with whom they can form a meaningful relationship.

52. A student asks the instructor about the difference between schizophrenia and Schizoid Personality Disorder. An appropriate response by the instructor would be that individuals with Schizoid Personality Disorder

    1. have almost all the cognitive attributes of schizophrenia.

    2. resemble anxious people.

    3. appear as just plain odd.

    4. have long periods of normal behavior interrupted by periods of Schizoid Personality Disorder.

53. A client's wife asks the nurse about the difference between Paranoid Personality Disorder and paranoid schizophrenia. The most appropriate response by the nurse would be which of the following?

    1. People with Paranoid Personality Disorder can lash out violently toward a person who makes them feel threatened, whereas people with schizophrenia are unlikely to be violent when provoked by acute feelings of paranoia toward a person.

    2. People with Paranoid Personality Disorder are more likely to experience hallucinations, whereas people with schizophrenia of the paranoid type are more likely to have delusions.

    3. People with schizophrenia of the paranoid type are psychotic, whereas people with Paranoid Personality Disorder are not likely to be psychotic.

    4. People with schizophrenia of the paranoid type are likely to be paranoid all the time, whereas people with Paranoid Personality Disorder are likely to be paranoid only occasionally.

54. The best nursing approach toward clients with odd or eccentric personality disorders is to

    1. draw the clients' attention to the cognitive aspects of their disorders.

    2. focus on relationship building.

    3. minimize or dismiss disturbing or bizarre thoughts.

    4. give the clients feedback on their behavior.

55. Compared to Obsessive-Compulsive Disorder (OCD), Obsessive-Compulsive Personality Disorder (OCPD)

    1. involves behavior in response to highly specific stimuli.

    2. is a pervasive disorder that encompasses every aspect of its victims' life.

    3. tends to disappear toward midlife.

    4. sufferers have more insight into their disorder than people suffering from OCD.

56. A client is diagnosed with Avoidant Personality Disorder. The nurse recognizes that the client will most likely try to avoid

    1. anything that would tend to raise the person's visibility.

    2. responsibility.

    3. immediate family members and close friends.

    4. familiar surroundings.

57. In planning for a client diagnosed with a Dependent Personality Disorder, the nurse recognizes these clients demonstrate not only the need to be cared for by others, but also

    1. indecisiveness.

    2. strong opinions.

    3. unusual maturity.

    4. highly risky behavior.

58. Another name for Passive-Aggressive Personality Disorder is

    1. Maddening Personality Disorder.

    2. Negativistic Personality Disorder.

    3. Antisocial Personality Disorder.

    4. Mother-in-Law Syndrome.

59. In planning care for clients with personality disorders, the nurse must keep in mind that

    1. we all have these disorders sooner or later.

    2. these are extremely common disorders affecting a large percentage of the population.

    3. personality disorders are highly treatable.

    4. personality disorders are characterized by pervasive personality traits that seriously impair their victims' ability to function.

60. Research shows that nurses respond least empathically to clients who are diagnosed with

    1. Borderline Personality Disorder.

    2. Antisocial Personality Disorder.

    3. schizophrenia.

    4. Bipolar Disorder.

61. In planning care for clients with somatization disorders, the nurse recognizes that these clients

    1. have a physical disease and don't know it.

    2. don't have a physical disease and don't know it.

    3. have a physical disease and know it.

    4. don't have a physical disease but are convinced they do.

62. In developing a treatment plan using cognitive-behavioral therapy, what do nurses recognize as the leading obstacle to its effectiveness with clients experiencing a somatization disorder?

    1. It usually only works in combination with medication therapy.

    2. "Cures" of physical disabilities are greeted with skepticism.

    3. It can take years for improvements.

    4. Clients won't accept it because they don't believe there is a psychological component to their illness.

63. The best approach for nurses to take toward people with hypochondriasis is to

    1. ignore the clients' concerns about their physical health and concentrate on psychosocial issues, as with other psychiatric disorders in which clients imagine fears not based on reality.

    2. recommend an intensive physical work-up.

    3. emphasize the clients' general good health and put symptoms in the context of being real and troublesome, not imaginary or dangerous.

    4. identify any other psychiatric disorder the clients may have and focus on the alternate diagnosis.

64. When planning a lecture on the key difference between conversion reaction and a Factitious Disorder, the instructor would include the fact that

    1. the cause of conversion reaction is psychological, whereas the source of Factitious Disorder is antisocial.

    2. the cause of conversion reaction is physical, whereas the source of Factitious Disorder is psychological.

    3. conversion reaction is a somatoform disorder, whereas Factitious Disorder arises from personality disorders.

    4. people with conversion reaction believe they are physically ill, whereas people with Factitious Disorder know deep down inside that they are not.

65. A nurse is caring for a client with Factitious Disorder. An appropriate intervention would be to

    1. help the clients recognize that, with current limitations on the resources of the health care system, health professionals cannot be squandering these resources on people who feign illness.

    2. recognize that, in their own unique way, people with Factitious Disorder are as much in need of psychiatric care as people with other psychiatric disorders.

    3. redirect those who feign illness to practitioners who feign cures.

    4. recommend vigorous interventions to satisfy clients who present themselves as ill.

66. A client asks the nurse if his primary insomnia is a mental disorder. The most appropriate response by the nurse would be that primary insomnia is only considered a psychiatric disorder if

    1. it lasts a month and interferes with a person's functioning.

    2. it is a consequence of some other psychiatric disorder.

    3. it has an organic cause.

    4. the client defines it as a psychiatric disorder.

67. Nurses can teach clients to improve sleep hygiene by recommending that they

    1. restrict the bedroom to sleep and sexual activity only.

    2. eat a heavy meal before retiring.

    3. have an alcoholic beverage before retiring.

    4. rise when the sun rises and retire when the sun sets.

68. A client is diagnosed with narcolepsy. The nurse recognizes that narcolepsy is

    1. the opposite of sleepwalking.

    2. a side effect of addiction to narcotics.

    3. a rare disorder that may run in families, characterized by sleep attacks accompanied by cataplexy or hallucinations.

    4. a fictitious disorder made up by writers.

69. A client asks the nurse about the key difference between nightmares and sleep terrors. Which of the following responses by the nurse is *not* correct?

    1. Nightmare Disorder is a DSM-IV-TR diagnosis, whereas there is no such DSM-IV-TR disorder as sleep terror disorder.

    2. Clients can remember the content of nightmares but they cannot remember the content of sleep terrors.

    3. Nightmares often require an extensive diagnostic work-up in a sleep disorders clinic, whereas the diagnosis of sleep terrors is relatively straightforward.

    4. They are the same things.

70. Developing a positive body image is important to adolescents. Nurses can promote a positive body image by teaching adolescents the "Three A's." Of the following, which is *not* considered part of the Three A's?

    1. Accept yourself for what you are.

    2. Attention: Feed, rest, and exercise your body based on the cues it gives you.

    3. Apprehension or Alarm: Be able to recognize when your body is getting too fat.

    4. Appreciation: Enjoy your body for the pleasure and safety it provides.

71. The mother of a client diagnosed with an eating disorder asks the nurse about the key difference between Bulimia Nervosa and Anorexia Nervosa. The nurse would be correct in responding that

    1. people with anorexia have a distorted body image that impels them to continue losing weight to a point where their body develops dangerous medical conditions; people with bulimia just use bingeing and purging as a dysfunctional means of weight control.

    2. bulimia is generally treated outside the hospital; once the client is admitted to the hospital for treatment, the diagnosis becomes anorexia.

    3. people with bulimia use fasting, bingeing, and purging as means of weight control; people with anorexia use fasting and exercising.

    4. bulimia is episodic, whereas anorexia is a long-term diagnosis.

72. A client is diagnosed with Hypoactive Sexual Desire Disorder. The nurse recognizes that this disorder is most frequently caused by

    1. advancing age.

    2. hormonal abnormalities.

    3. relationship problems.

    4. gender identity problems.

73. A nurse is preparing a presentation on sexuality and gender identity. The nurse's presentation would include that according to the DSM-IV-TR, which of the following is not considered a disorder of sexuality and gender identity?

    1. Homosexuality

    2. Gender identity

    3. Premature ejaculation

    4. Exhibitionism

74. Knowledge and skills necessary for nurses to effectively manage pain in their clients include all of the following except

    1. political and administrative skills to ensure that clients receive the best possible care.

    2. advanced practice certification.

    3. knowledge of pharmacology.

    4. knowledge of the neurobiology of pain.

75. The main role of the liaison psychiatric nurse is to

    1. keep the psychiatrist informed of his or her clients' developments while they are hospitalized for physical conditions.

    2. provide consultation and teaching to medical nurses when a client with a psychiatric condition is being treated in a medical unit.

    3. handle the questions from clients' families.

    4. provide psychiatric care to clients who are physically ill.

76. Psychoneuroimmunology is a field that seeks to

    1. find the physical causes of stress.

    2. understand the biological basis for mental illnesses.

    3. understand the mind-body connection.

    4. find ways to boost the body's ability to withstand stress.

77. All of the following contributed to massive deinstitutionalization of people with chronic or severe mental illnesses in the late 1960s and 1970s except

    1. concern for the civil rights of people with mental illnesses.

    2. desire for cost cutting.

    3. full commitment to mental health treatment and support services in the community.

    4. significant improvements in the medications available to treat mental disorders.

78. Just as there are "childhood" diseases among the physical diseases, there are also "childhood" disorders among the mental illnesses. Mental disorders unique to childhood include all of the following except

    1. personality disorders.

    2. Autistic Disorder.

    3. Conduct Disorder.

    4. Attention-Deficit Hyperactivity Disorder.

79. Nurses should be alert to the following dynamics of childhood depression except which?

    1. Many traditional clinicians don't believe children experience depression.

    2. Childhood depression may manifest itself as irritable or aggressive behavior.

    3. Depressed children become delusional.

    4. Depression in children may be related to neglect or abuse.

80. All of the following nursing skills are useful in assessing the mental health of a child except

    1. family assessment skills.

    2. play therapy.

    3. developmental assessment knowledge.

    4. psychodrama.

81. Asperger's Syndrome differs from autism in that

    1. Asperger's does not lead to social isolation.

    2. Asperger's is treatable.

    3. Asperger's is characterized by repetitive actions or behaviors.

    4. Asperger's is associated with no known neurological abnormalities.

82. When working with adolescents, a school nurse recognizes that which of the following is the healthiest form of identity formation?

    1. Identity achievement

    2. Foreclosure

    3. Moratorium

    4. Identity diffusion

83. Adolescence is an age group at high risk for suicide. Signs that should raise concerns about an increased risk for suicide include all of the following except

    1. an increase in impulsive behavior.

    2. giving away cherished belongings.

    3. decreased appetite.

    4. preoccupation with death and dying.

84. When working with a group of adolescents, the school nurse hypothesizes that the factor that most protects teenagers from engaging in dangerous risk-taking behaviors is

    1. an authoritarian parenting style.

    2. connectedness with parents and school.

    3. strong spiritual beliefs.

    4. their peer group.

85. Of the following, which is *not* an action that nurses can take to help develop a therapeutic relationship with an adolescent?

    1. Understand interests and lifestyle choices currently popular with adolescents.

    2. Self-disclose information as a means of validating an adolescent's experience.

    3. Help adolescents identify their strengths and reasons for positive self-image.

    4. Listen actively.

86. A nurse caring for clients with dementia would most likely find all of the following signs and symptoms except

    1. paranoia.

    2. disinhibition.

    3. wandering.

    4. reminiscing.

87. Ways nurses can assist fatigued caretakers of elderly friends and relatives with dementia include

    1. suggesting clients' physicians order or increase sedatives.

    2. assisting caregivers in planning alternate care arrangements in a guilt-free manner consistent with the clients' best interests.

    3. encouraging caregivers to discuss their fatigue frankly with clients.

    4. helping caregivers accept their fatigue and stress.

88. Nurses are obligated to take action in response to a client who is the victim of child abuse or rape. Of the following, which is *not* considered an action that nurses should take?

    1. Nurses must report child abuse or rape to the appropriate authorities.

    2. Nurses should know how to maintain the integrity of any evidence needed to prosecute a crime.

    3. Nurses should understand the dynamics of abuse and examine their own feelings toward these issues.

    4. Nurses should treat these cases like any other physical injury that has psychosocial implications.

89. Atypical neuroleptics are gaining wide acceptance in the treatment of psychosis because they are

    1. cheaper than haloperidol and other phenathiazines.

    2. preferred by clients who want the latest treatments.

    3. safe for children under 18.

    4. relatively free of extra-pyramidal side effects.

90. Prescribing stimulants is controversial because these drugs are easily abused and their effectiveness is either unproven or heatedly debated, except for the treatment of

    1. Attention-Deficit Disorder.

    2. anxiety.

    3. Obsessive-Compulsive Personality Disorder.

    4. narcolepsy.

91. A nursing instructor evaluates that further teaching is necessary if a student responds that psychoanalysis

    1. remains useful today.

    2. is an expensive, lengthy form of therapy that insurance does not usually cover and few individuals can afford.

    3. is only effective in treating schizophrenia.

    4. has given way to shorter, more cost-effective forms of individual therapy.

92. An Advance Practice Nurse would plan to use cognitive-behavioral therapy because this form of therapy

    1. offers insight into the childhood origins of adult problems.

    2. works by allowing clients to "talk through" their problems.

    3. offers solutions to problems that actively involve making behavioral changes.

    4. is similar to psychoanalysis in the cost and length of treatment.

93. Nurses find it useful to view families as systems because

    1. families are less than the sum of their parts (individuals).

    2. dysfunctions cannot produce equilibria.

    3. the changes affecting an individual have an effect on the whole family.

    4. other parts of society work like systems.

94. The *trifocal model* refers to

    1. individual, family, and community.

    2. wellness, prevention, and problem intervention.

    3. medicine, nursing, and allied health.

    4. id, ego, and superego.

95. When a nursing diagnosis of Caregiver Role Strain has been established, it is important for the nurse to

    1. give the stressed caregiver regular breaks.

    2. teach the caregiver more about caring models.

    3. recognize the ways in which the caregiver adds to his or her own strain.

    4. include the caregiver in the health care planning team.

96. Ecomaps are a useful way to

    1. assess the genetic component of diseases in the family.

    2. identify the person in the family with the greatest psychic strength.

    3. understand family dynamics.

    4. develop nursing care plans.

97. An Advance Practice Nurse Therapist would encourage clients to participate in group therapy because this form of therapy is an excellent way to

    1. get withdrawn clients to talk.

    2. make clients feel that they are not alone, that others share their problems.

    3. get better compliance on the unit, due to the collaborative decision making.

    4. elicit extremely personal revelations.

98. When evaluating a student's knowledge of health care financing, the instructor determines that learning has occurred if the student states that capitation

    1. cuts off claimants.

    2. establishes a single payment for a particular kind of disorder, like mental disorders, for a specific period of time to limit the insurer's liability.

    3. identifies coverages or clients the insurance company won't cover.

    4. charges a "per head" fee for services as they are delivered.

99. Relaxation techniques and guided imagery are examples of treatment modalities that are

    1. complementary, or adjunct, to other psychiatric treatment modalities.

    2. inappropriate to nursing practice.

    3. not proven to be ineffective.

    4. harmful, not helpful.

100. Centering is a nursing self-care modality that

    1. once learned, takes only 30 to 60 seconds to perform.

    2. helps the nurse focus on the work immediately ahead.

    3. releases tension, placing the nurse fully in the present.

    4. encompasses all of the above.

ANSWERS TO SELF-ASSESSMENT QUIZZES

Chapter 1:
Through the Door: Your First Day in Psychiatric Nursing

1. b
2. c
3. d
4. a
5. c
6. c
7. b
8. b
9. b
10. c
11. c
12. *Rites of passage* might be defined as experiences that mark a significant event, achievement, pathway, or growth.
13. *Being present* could be defined as caring, listening, affirming, and responding to or supporting clients, often in nurturing, nonverbal ways.

Chapter 2:
Psychiatric Nursing: Evolution of a Specialty

1. a
2. a
3. b
4. a
5. c
6. a
7. c
8. b, a, d, g, e, c, f
9. f, g, a, d, b, c, e

Chapter 3:
Theory as a Basis for Practice

1. Relationships
2. Modeling
3. Leininger, Watson, and/or Boyken & Schoenhofer
4. Energy Fields
5. Self-Care Deficit
6. Id, ego, and superego
7. Erikson
8. Social or interpersonal
9. Cognitive
10. Behavioral
11. a
12. c
13. a

14. c

15. a

16. b

17. c

Chapter 4:
Neuroscience as a Basis for Practice

1. d

2. c

3. a

4. c

5. c

6. b

7. b

8. a

9. b

10. b

11. c

12. a

Chapter 5:
Diagnostic Systems for Psychiatric Nursing

1. c

2. b

3. d

4. a

5. a

Chapter 6:
Tools of Psychiatric Mental Health Nursing: Communication, Nursing Process, and the Nurse-Client Relationship

1. d

2. d

3. c

4. d

5. d

6. d

7. c

8. b

9. c

10. a

11. d

12. c

13. a

14. c

15. b

16. d

Chapter 7:
Cultural and Ethnic Considerations

1. a

2. d

3. a

4. c

5. b

6. a

7. c

8. d

9. b

10. a

11. c, a, b, f, d, e

Chapter 8:
Epidemiology of Mental Health Illness

1. c

2. b

3. a

4. d

5. c

6. f

7. c

8. a

9. b

10. d

Chapter 9:
Ethical and Legal Bases for Care

1. c

2. a

3. b

4. b

5. a

6. a

7. c

8. a

9. c

10. b

Chapter 10:
Self-Care for the Nurse

1. c

2. d

3. d

4. c

5. c

6. d

7. b

8. c

9. c

10. a

Chapter 11:
The Client Undergoing Crisis

1. b

2. a

3. d

4. d

5. c

6. c

7. c

8. d

9. c

10. b

Chapter 12:
The Client Experiencing Anxiety

1. b
2. a
3. c
4. b
5. c
6. c
7. d
8. a
9. c

Chapter 13:
The Client Experiencing Schizophrenia

1. d
2. c and f
3. c
4. b
5. b
6. a
7. c
8. d
9. b

Chapter 14:
The Client Experiencing Depression

1. c
2. d
3. a
4. a
5. b
6. a

7. b
8. c
9. d
10. a
11. b
12. T, T, M, S, T, M, S, T, S, T

Chapter 15:
The Client Experiencing Mania

1. b
2. a
3. a
4. d
5. c
6. b
7. a
8. d
9. c
10. c
11. c
12. a
13. d

Chapter 16:
The Client Who Is Suicidal

1. d
2. b
3. d
4. c
5. b
6. a
7. a

8. a

9. a

10. d

Chapter 17:
The Client Who Abuses Chemical Substances

1. c

2. b

3. a

4. c

5. d

6. c

7. c

8. c

9. f

10. d

Chapter 18:
The Client with a Personality Disorder

1. c

2. b

3. d

4. c

5. a

6. d

7. c

8. a

9. c

10. d

Chapter 19:
The Client Experiencing a Somatoform, Factitious, or Dissociative Disorder

1. b

2. a

3. c

4. b

5. a

6. d

7. c

8. c

9. e

10. c

Chapter 20:
The Client with Disorders of Self-Regulation: Sleep Disorders, Eating Disorders, and Sexual Disorders

1. a

2. d

3. c

4. c

5. b

6. a

7. g

8. a

9. c

10. d

Chapter 21:
The Physically Ill Client
Experiencing Emotional Distress

1. c
2. a
3. c
4. b
5. d
6. c
7. a
8. c
9. c
10. b

Chapter 22:
Forgotten Populations: The Homeless and the Incarcerated

1. a
2. b
3. c
4. d

Chapter 23:
The Child

1. c
2. c
3. d
4. b
5. a
6. b
7. a
8. c
9. b

10. a
11. a

Chapter 24:
The Adolescent

1. a
2. d
3. b
4. c
5. d
6. c
7. b
8. c
9. a
10. a
11. b

Chapter 25:
The Elderly

1. b
2. c
3. d
4. d
5. a
6. a
7. b
8. c
9. a
10. a

Chapter 26:
Violence: An Issue for Psychiatric Mental Health Nursing

1. c

2. b

3. a

4. a

5. a

Chapter 27:
Pharmacology in Psychiatric Care

1. c

2. a

3. b

4. d

5. a

6. d

7. c

8. d

9. b

10. c

11. b

12. P

    D

    P

    A

    A

    A

    P

    D

    D

P

A

P

A

P

Chapter 28:
Individual Psychotherapy

1. c

2. d

3. a

4. c

5. b

6. b

7. a

8. c

9. a

10. c

Chapter 29:
Family Therapy

1. b

2. a

3. c

4. b

5. b

6. d

7. c

8. a

9. c

10. b

Chapter 30:
Group Therapy

1. a
2. a
3. c
4. b
5. c
6. d
7. b
8. a
9. c
10. c

Chapter 31:
Community Mental Health Nursing

1. b
2. a
3. b
4. b

5. c
6. c
7. d
8. b
9. b
10. b

Chapter 32:
Complementary and Somatic Therapies

1. b
2. a
3. a
4. c
5. b
6. a
7. b
8. c
9. c
10. a

ANSWERS AND RATIONALES TO COMPREHENSIVE NCLEX STYLE PRACTICE FINAL EXAMINATION

1. **Answer: 2.**

   Neurotransmitters are the chemical messengers released across the synaptic cleft. The dendrites then respond to the message in an inhibitory or excitatory manner. Neurotransmitters act in either an inhibitory or excitatory manner. When acting in an inhibitory manner, activity is decreased. When excited, activity increases.

2. **Answer: 3.**

   The current revision of the Diagnostic Statistical Manual is the DSM-IV-TR. This revision alerts the clinician to gather information related to a culturally sensitive assessment. Information gathered includes the cultural identity of the individual, cultural explanations of the individual's illness, cultural factors related to psychosocial environment and levels of functioning, cultural elements of the relationship between the individual and the child, and an overall cultural assessment for diagnosis and care.

3. **Answer: 3.**

   Axis IV of the Diagnostic Statistical Manual identifies psychosocial and environmental problems. Axis I identifies clinical psychiatric disorders, Axis III identifies general medical disorders, and Axis V identifies global assessment of functioning.

4. **Answer: 1.**

   Surprisingly, more than half of the approved/accepted nursing diagnoses address nursing concerns in the psychosocial-spiritual realm of client care. This fact underscores that the essence of nursing includes meeting the mental health, emotional, and spiritual needs of clients.

5. **Answer: 4**.

Defense mechanisms are unconscious responses used by persons to protect themselves from internal conflicts and external stress. When a nurse concludes that the client is using a defense mechanism to avoid dealing with certain subjects, the nurse can use this knowledge to guide interactions, knowing that the defense mechanism indicates the presence of psychologically significant material.

6. **Answer: 3**.

The Carter Commission identified the prevalence and incidence of mental illness. The tip-of-the-iceberg phenomenon was based on the Sterling County Study. The Community Mental Health Centers Act promoted deinstitutionalization, and the Brown Report recommended that psychiatric nursing become part of general nursing education.

7. **Answer: 3**.

Clients admitted to a psychiatric unit retain the right to receive and refuse treatment. They also retain the right to informed consent and the right to control personal affairs. However, they lose the right of free will to leave the hospital at any time. In addition, they do not have the right to smoke, disrupt treatment of other clients, or be judged by a panel of their peers.

8. **Answer: 1**.

Nurses are obligated to use the least restrictive alternative. Such a method may include one-to-one supervision. The principle is a legal doctrine that requires that clients be treated with the least amount of constraint of liberty consistent with their safety.

9. **Answer: 3**.

Selye's General Adaptation Syndrome is a model of a human being's healthy response to stress and includes three major stages. The individual's initial response involves an alarm reaction, then a stage of resistance, and a final stage of exhaustion. The first and third stages are broken down further to include shock and countershock.

10. **Answer: 3**.

The key difference between fear and anxiety is that fear is a response triggered by a known, specific object which produces an autonomic response. A person experiencing anxiety would have a sense of dread without having a specific source or reason for the emotion.

11. **Answer: 2.**

Nurses caring for individuals who experience Panic Disorder should help the client cognitively reframe the stressful situation. Providing false reassurance is inappropriate. Sedation will not facilitate problem solving and the client may not be able to concentrate enough to meditate.

12. **Answer: 3.**

Panic Disorder is a form of anxiety. The person has feelings of dread or terror and is unable to control his or her behavior. The individual will experience a sense of awe, possibly losing control and becoming disorganized.

13. **Answer: 4.**

Obsessive-Compulsive Disorder is an appropriate diagnosis when fear of self-contamination is inconsistent with the risk. Obsessions in Obsessive-Compulsive Disorder are recurrent thoughts, images, or impulses that are experienced as intrusive and inappropriate. The obsessions cause marked anxiety or distress which is only relieved by performing a compulsive act. Compulsions are repetitive behaviors or acts such as constantly washing hands. The compulsions serve as a method of reducing the anxiety which the person experiences from the obsessive thoughts.

14. **Answer: 2.**

It is important for the nurse to identify if the client uses alcohol or not. The choice of treatment for the anxiety will be based on whether the focus is to help the individual achieve insight or whether behaviors should be changed to reduce the anxiety. In addition, certain medications react negatively with alcohol.

15. **Answer: 2.**

The nurse would recognize that the client is using word salad. Word salad is speech marked by a group of disconnected words.

16. **Answer: 1.**

The positive symptoms of schizophrenia include hallucinations, delusions, and disordered thinking. Flat affect, lack of relationships, poverty of speech, lack of motivation, and symptoms of depression are examples of negative symptoms of schizophrenia.

17. **Answer: 3**.

The negative symptoms of schizophrenia include anhedonia, flattened affect, poverty of speech, and other symptoms of depression. The other options listed are positive symptoms of schizophrenia.

18. **Answer: 2**.

The dopamine hypothesis postulates that functional abnormalities in schizophrenia are due to excessive activity of brain dopamine. Dopamine is normally produced in the brain, and it serves as a signaling molecule or neurotransmitter. Dopamine seems to have the most important effects in the basal ganglia of the brain.

19. **Answer: 3**.

Medications are the only treatment for schizophrenia that have been proven. Some evidence does suggest that electroconvulsive therapy may be of value to selective clients in catatonic states, when used in association with antipsychotic medication. However, the benefits are sometimes only short term.

20. **Answer: 1**.

The priority action is for the nurse to redirect the conversation back to reality. The nurse should never ask the client to tell her more, enter into the delusion, or argue with the client over the reality of the delusion. Speaking louder is not an appropriate response because the voices the client hears (the hallucinations) are internal and not external to the client.

21. **Answer: 3**.

During the rehabilitative phase of schizophrenia, the nurse should help clients structure their day with a written schedule. The other options are not nursing actions appropriate for the rehabilitative phase.

22. **Answer: 3**.

The major difference between unipolar and bipolar depression is that the client with bipolar depression has upswings or highs at least some of the time.

23. **Answer: 3**.

A major symptom of Major Depressive Disorder involves suicidal thoughts. These thoughts place the client at risk for self-harm. Grandiosity is characteristic of thought disorders, not mood disorders such as Major Depression.

24. **Answer: 2**.

The family should be taught that for an individual to be diagnosed with a dysthymic mood disorder, a person must experience a depressed mood for at least 2 years. The individual feels depressed nearly all of the time. The depressed mood is experienced most of the day, for more days than not. A person with Dysthymic Disorder must also have at least two of the following symptoms: appetite disturbance, sleep disturbance, fatigue, low self-esteem, poor concentration or difficulty making decisions, and feelings of hopelessness.

25. **Answer: 3**.

The normal stages of grief include shock, reality, and recovery. Chronic grief is not normal. It is an example of dysfunctional grief.

26. **Answer: 1**.

According to Sigmund Freud's psychoanalytic perspective, the superego is an inner voice or conscience. For example, in depression, the superego punishes the ego for having forbidden wishes or for not living up to the superego's expectations (usually similar to those of one's actual parents). The result of that conflict is guilt, self-hate, and anger turned inward; these processes in turn lead to depression.

27. **Answer: 2**.

The pharmacologic treatment of depression includes the use of antidepressant medications such as tricyclics, selective serotonin reuptake inhibitors (SSRIs), and monoamine oxidase inhibitors (MAOIs). Phenothiazines are most often used in schizophrenia but can be used with clients with Bipolar Disorder. Phenothiazines are used for the thought disorders present in these conditions.

28. **Answer: 4**.

According to Orem's Self-Care Deficit Theory of Nursing, encouraging the client to meet his or her own needs increases the client's sense of self-care agency. The concept of nursing agency refers to nursing activities required to compensate for the client's inability to meet his or her own self-care requirements. Nurses who base their care on Orem's theory must plan care carefully and determine what and when the client can do for self and when nursing actions are necessary.

29. **Answer: 1.**

The nurse should inform the client's husband that the defining characteristics of hypomania include the same seven criteria for mania, but to diagnose hypomania, only three symptoms need to be present. These three symptoms need only have lasted 4 days. In contrast to mania, hypomanic symptoms need not cause any disturbances in functioning but must be observable by others.

30. **Answer: 3.**

The transition from mania to depression or depression to mania is called the *switch process*. Individuals who experience this switch several times are known as *rapid cyclers* because they switch from episodes of euphoria to episodes of depression. Rapid cyclers are defined as individuals who have four or more episodes in a year. Although the overall incidence of Bipolar Disorder does not differ much between men and women, nearly all rapid cyclers are women.

31. **Answer: 1.**

There is strong evidence to suggest that Bipolar Disorder is caused by genetic factors, meaning there is a tendency for this disorder to be inherited. Some of the best data on the inheritance of manic-depressive illness come from studies of twins. If one of two identical twins is manic-depressive, the other is almost certain to develop the disease. For fraternal twins (who share much less of their genetic makeup), the risk is much lower, about 20%.

32. **Answer: 4.**

Drugs, physical diseases, and sleep disruptions can all produce symptoms similar to mania. Financial difficulties are more likely to cause symptoms of depression.

33. **Answer: 2.**

Lithium, tricyclic antidepressants, and St. John's wort can cause switching from depressive episodes to a manic state. However, anabolic steroids will not cause this reaction.

34. **Answer: 1.**

Further teaching is needed if the client responds that Lithium is ineffective in eliminating mood swings because eliminating mood swings is a major action of this medication. The other options are correct statements about Lithium.

35. **Answer: 3.**

The primary treatment for Bipolar Disorder is medication such as Lithium. Psychotherapy and behavior therapy may be used, but they are not major forms of treatment.

36. **Answer: 4.**

The priority nursing intervention for this client would be to provide a structured, nonstimulating environment. The environment should be free of objects that could be used to harm self or others and free of extraneous noise or stimulation. All verbal communication from the nurse should be short, concise, and clear. The client must be assisted with developing a slower pace than the one he or she has been experiencing over the past 2 weeks.

37. **Answer: 3.**

An example of tertiary prevention of suicide might be learning CPR and other emergency medical procedures. Tertiary prevention in the area of suicide is best represented by an increase in survival rates of persons attempting suicide. Tertiary prevention focuses on rehabilitation and restoration.

38. **Answer: 2.**

The nurse can reduce the risk of suicide attempts by the client by having the client sign a written no-suicide contract. Most therapists agree that when clients readily agree to not harm themselves during a prescribed period, risk is decreased. Often such contracts are written and signed, and the client is assured he or she has someone to call if he or she cannot bear it alone.

39. **Answer: 4.**

Clients diagnosed with drug dependence often try unsuccessfully to stop using a substance. This results in the need for treatment in a formal and professionally supervised treatment program.

40. **Answer: 3.**

The CAGE questionnaire is normally used to detect alcoholism. It is not appropriate to use the CAGE questionnaire to detect claustrophobia or mania, or for determining abuse of substances other than alcohol.

41. **Answer: 1.**

Opiates are powerfully addicting substances because they fit perfectly into endorphin receptors. They provide a pleasurable and euphoric feeling when used.

42. **Answer: 1**.

   Methadone prevents withdrawal symptoms while blocking the pleasurable affects of opiates, allowing the client to function without drug euphoria.

43. **Answer: 4**.

   The nurse should teach teens that the major danger with using hallucinogens is that the individual never returns to normal. Flashbacks of the experience often return at a later date.

44. **Answer: 1**.

   Up to 50% of people who abuse drugs abuse more than one drug and/or have another psychiatric disorder.

45. **Answer: 3**.

   Codependence refers to the relationship between a substance abuser and a significant other who facilitates the substance use. An example of codependence is calling in to a spouse's workplace to report that he or she has the flu when he or she is sick from drugging. The spouse who calls the workplace is acting in the codependent role. *Codependence* is a term used to describe the cluster of behaviors exhibited by family members/significant others (most often a spouse) of one who is chemically addicted that serve to enable the alcoholic or addict to continue using the substance. Codependent behaviors serve to satisfy the needs of the family member to feel loved, important, and needed.

46. **Answer: 3**.

   Personality disorders are generally diagnosed in adolescence and adulthood. The majority of individuals diagnosed with Borderline Personality Disorder are women in their teens and twenties.

47. **Answer: 4**.

   Personality disorders are classified as Axis II disorders in the DSM-IV-TR because major psychiatric disorders on Axis I are constant across all personality types and Axis II disorders color Axis I disorders.

48. **Answer: 3**.

   Antisocial personality disorders are considered in the "dramatic and emotional group" of disorders.

49. **Answer: 3**.

The term *borderline* refers to the client living on the border between psychosis and neurosis.

50. **Answer: 3**.

The nurse recognizes that these clients have difficulty dealing with life stressors. Males are more likely to develop Narcissistic Personality Disorder. The developmental history of persons with Narcissistic Personality Disorder typically shows a pattern of selfless love and adoration from a significant adult. At the same time, the child experiences an ever-present threat of criticism for not being perfect. As adults, they appear arrogant, conceited, insensitive, and ruthless. While the personality structure is stable, it is very rigid.

51. **Answer: 3**.

Individuals with Antisocial Personality Disorder often view the nurse as a means to an end, like everybody else in their lives.

52. **Answer: 3**.

"Eccentric" is the most appropriate descriptor of a person with Schizotypal Personality Disorder. Such individuals have great difficulty forming close relationships with others, and therefore would not likely be referred to as "warm." They are not known to be particularly jovial. Other terms used to describe a person with Schizotypal Personality Disorder are "odd" and "peculiar."

53. **Answer: 3**.

Individuals with schizophrenia of the paranoid type are psychotic, meaning they have lost touch with reality. On the other hand, individuals with Paranoid Personality Disorder are not likely to be psychotic, but have a definite flaw in their personalities.

54. **Answer: 4**.

The best nursing approach toward clients with odd or eccentric personality disorders is to give the client feedback on his behavior. The nurse should give the client realistic feedback on why the person is not being understood. The nurse can be most helpful in providing measured feedback to the client regarding behavior and statements. This will help the client learn to adjust the behaviors that may be causing him difficulty in life. A common theme is that these individuals experience an inability to establish and maintain close interpersonal relationships.

55. **Answer: 2.**

The diagnosis for OCPD is distinct from OCD, although it shares the same rigid behaviors and patterns, such as hoarding personal effects or other items. As OCD is an anxiety disorder and not a personality disorder, an individual suffering from it is typically normal psychologically, except in situations which provoke their obsessions. In contrast, the rigidity displayed by a person suffering from OCPD is generally more extreme and more pervasive. It is not limited to a few specific stressors/compulsions.

56. **Answer: 1.**

Individuals with Avoidant Personality Disorder try to avoid anything that would tend to raise their visibility. The major features of this disorder include social inhibition and feelings of inadequacy. These individuals tend to avoid interpersonal situations at work or school that could lead to criticism or rejection.

57. **Answer: 1.**

Characteristics of clients with Dependent Personality Disorder include the need to be cared for by others. They exhibit indecisiveness and difficulty expressing disagreement with others. These individuals are submissive and fear separation from the known.

58. **Answer: 2.**

Passive-Aggressive Personality Disorder is also known as Negativistic Personality Disorder. Individuals with this disorder have a negative outlook on life. They tend to be sullen, irritable, impatient, argumentative, cynical, skeptical, and contrary. They often feel cheated, unappreciated, and misunderstood.

59. **Answer: 4.**

Regardless of the type of personality disorder, these disorders are characterized by pervasive personality traits that seriously impair their victims' ability to function. Personality disorders generally lead to distress. They are pervasive and inflexible, have their onset in adolescence or early adulthood, and are stable over time. Personality disorders do not resolve in midlife.

60. **Answer: 1.**

Research has shown that nurses respond least empathetically to clients who are diagnosed with Borderline Personality Disorder.

61. **Answer: 4**.

Somatoform disorders are a group of conditions in which symptoms suggest the presence of a general medical condition, but careful evaluation fails to find any evidence of a physical disorder sufficient to explain the complaints. Most experts feel that psychological factors account for the symptoms of somatoform disorders. Clients with this disorder truly feel they have a physical illness.

62. **Answer: 4**.

One of the major problems with treating clients with somatoform disorders is their failure to keep appointments with a psychotherapist. Many of the clients do not believe they are psychologically ill. They seek different medical opinions in order to verify that they have a physical problem.

63. **Answer: 3**.

The best approach for nurses to take toward people with Hypochondriasis is to emphasize the client's general good health and put symptoms in the context of being real and troublesome, not imaginary or dangerous.

64. **Answer: 4**.

The key difference between conversion reaction and Factitious Disorder is that people with conversion reaction believe they are ill, whereas people with Factitious Disorder know deep down inside that they are not. Individuals with acute conversion often respond to direct explanation of the psychological conflicts the individual is experiencing. However, individuals with Factitious Disorder report physical or psychological symptoms that are intentionally produced in order to gain attention from potential caregivers.

65. **Answer: 2**.

An appropriate response to people with Factitious Disorder is to recognize that in their own unique way, these individuals are as much in need of psychiatric care as people with other psychiatric disorders.

66. **Answer: 1**.

Primary insomnia is considered a psychiatric disorder if it lasts a month and interferes with a person's functioning.

67. **Answer: 1**.

Nurses can teach clients to improve sleep hygiene by recommending that they restrict the bedroom to sleep and sexual activity only. Other interventions would include instructing the client to avoid foods other than warm milk within 3 to 4 hours of going to bed. While a light snack may help, a heavy meal will not.

68. **Answer: 3**.

Narcolepsy is a primary sleep disorder in which individuals frequently have three different and quite striking sleep-related symptoms. First, they have the frequent recurrence of an irresistible need for brief episodes of sleep. They awake from these episodes feeling remarkably refreshed and rarely report daytime sleepiness except immediately prior to one of these episodes. Second, narcoleptic persons often have vivid dreamlike states as they are falling asleep or waking up. Third, they may have episodes of cataplexy.

69. **Answer: 2**.

Sleep terrors are related to parasomnia in which there is no recall of the sleep-related event. Individuals experiencing sleep terrors rouse suddenly from sleep with a cry or scream. They typically sit up in bed in apparent terror; sweaty, pupils dilated, tachypneic, and tachycardic.

70. **Answer: 3**.

Self-concept disturbance is the most common psychological characteristic shared by both anorexics and bulimics. Specifically, both anorexics and bulimics have a distorted body image. In the case of anorexics, this distorted body image may cause individuals to see themselves as being fat, regardless of how thin or emaciated they become as a result of their disorder.

71. **Answer: 1**.

With anorexia nervosa, individuals actively starve themselves in an effort to keep from gaining weight. They engage in exercises which will cause weight loss. Fasting, binging, and purging are the three behaviors that represent the main aspects of bulimia nervosa. Typically, those engaging in bulimia nervosa hide their activities, and face a risk of being discovered by parents and/or other family members. Clients with bulimia tend to be a normal weight. On the other hand, clients with anorexia can become so emaciated as a result of starvation that there is a great risk of death. In such cases, forced feeding may be required because the client is unwilling, or physically unable, to feed himself or herself.

72. **Answer: 3**.

Hypoactive Sexual Desire Disorder is a disorder in which a person is evaluated as having a sex drive that is significantly lower than what would be normal for that individual. The client will usually report a distress or disturbance in interpersonal relationships. Relationship problems are the most frequent cause of Hypoactive Sexual Desire Disorder. However, the clinician should also inquire about physical conditions, affective disorders, and use of controlled substances, as these may also lead to a loss in sexual desire.

73. **Answer: 1**.

While homosexuality is certainly related to sexuality, it is no longer considered to be a mental disorder. As a result, it is not listed in the DSM-IV-TR. A psychiatric disorder requires that a person experience some degree of personal, vocational, or social dysfunction. One can be homosexual and not experience any of these things.

74. **Answer: 1**.

Political and administrative skills are not necessary for nurses to effectively manage pain in their clients. An understanding of the neurobiology of pain, as well as the physiological effects of the medications administered to the client, is more important. There are advanced practice certifications that go into great depth specifically in the area of pain management.

75. **Answer: 2**.

The role of the liaison nurse was developed in the 1960s for the purpose of serving as consultants for other health care providers. The liaison nurse role is one of two nursing roles which focus on treating clients who have strong emotional reactions to physical illnesses that they are currently suffering from. The second nursing role is the psychiatric nurse specialist in home care.

76. **Answer: 3**.

Psychoneuroimmunology is a branch of study that would best explain the mind-body connection. It is based on the theory of the relationships between psychological factors (emotions, feelings, thoughts, etc.) and the immune system. The immune system is influenced by these psychological factors through the hypothalamic pituitary axis of the sympathetic nervous system. This model is based on Selye's General Adaptation Syndrome.

77. **Answer: 3**.

There has never been a full commitment to mental health treatment and support services in the community. The push toward deinstitutionalization has been led by both civil rights advocates opposing the involuntary commitment of people diagnosed with mental disorders, as well as the realization that moving clients out of institutions and into the community could dramatically decrease the cost of caring for those clients. Also, pharmacological advances with regard to medications that treat mental disorders led to a decreased requirement for some clients to be constantly monitored in an institutionalized setting.

78. **Answer: 1**.

Personality disorders generally occur during adolescence and early adulthood. Common disorders of children include autism, Conduct Disorder, and Attention-Deficit Hyperactivity Disorder.

79. **Answer: 1**.

Virtually all clinicians believe that children can experience depression. Such depression in children may be the result of neglect or abuse. Irritable or aggressive behavior may be a symptom of childhood depression. Children suffering from depression may become delusional and, in some cases, suicidal.

80. **Answer: 4**.

Nurses assessing children for mental health problems would need skills related to play therapy, developmental assessment, and family assessment. Psychodrama is a form of treatment most often used with adults.

81. **Answer: 4**.

Children with Asperger's share many of the characteristics of autism, but are far less severely affected. Asperger's Syndrome is characterized by the combination of severe impairments in social interaction with highly repetitive patterns of interests and behaviors. These interests are often highly limited, but children with Asperger's frequently gain a great deal of knowledge about a relatively narrow range of topics. Unlike autism, where communication skills are severely impaired, children with Asperger's syndrome have normal repetitive and expressive language.

82. **Answer: 2**.

Foreclosure occurs when individuals have not thoroughly explored the possibilities of identity before making a commitment about adult status. They are closely tied to their families because questioning caregiver values would be too threatening and would make them feel guilty.

83. **Answer: 3**.

Adolescents at risk for suicide may exhibit behaviors such as an increase in impulsive behavior, preoccupation with death and dying, and giving away cherished belongings. A decrease in appetite is not specifically an indication of potential risk for suicide.

84. **Answer: 1**.

According to Jessor (1991), authoritarian caregivers provide clear boundaries and expectations for their children. As a result, the children of such caregivers, in general, engage in less risky behaviors, display greater psychosocial maturity, and perform better in school.

85. **Answer: 2**.

Self-disclosure by the nurse does not necessarily validate the adolescent's experience, but frequently satisfies the nurse's needs. It often interferes with the development of a therapeutic relationship by blurring the boundaries. More appropriate actions nurses can take to help develop a therapeutic relationship would include being nonjudgmental, active listening, understanding interests and lifestyle choices currently popular with adolescents, helping adolescents identify strengths, expressing positive feelings toward adolescents, and allowing adolescents to express their feelings openly.

86. **Answer: 4**.

Reminiscing is not a sign or symptom of dementia; it is a process by which an elderly person remembers and reviews experiences from the past. Paranoia, disinhibition, and wandering are characteristics seen in dementia.

87. **Answer: 2**.

The nurse can assist a fatigued caretaker by assisting the individual in planning alternative care arrangements. These arrangements may include identifying a temporary caregiver, day treatment programs, or short-term hospitalizations. These alternatives provide a form of respite for the caretaker.

88. **Answer: 4.**

The nurse is required by law to report all cases of suspected elder abuse to the proper authorities. The nurse is also obligated to report cases of child abuse.

89. **Answer: 4.**

Atypical (also known as "second-generation") antipsychotic medications are not uniform in how they work or what side effects they produce. The atypical antipsychotics have differing and often fewer side effects than the first-generation (also known as "classical") antipsychotic medications. In addition, they are frequently significantly more costly.

90. **Answer: 4.**

Stimulant medications have their best-documented use in the management of narcolepsy. They are effective in treating this disorder, which is characterized by daytime sleepiness. While stimulants are commonly used for Attention-Deficit Hyperactivity Disorder (ADHD), concern over their use has been expressed.

91. **Answer: 3**.

Psychoanalysis helps clients gain insight into how old unconscious factors affect current relationship and behavior patterns. The treatment traces the patterns of behavior and relationships back to their origin in infancy or childhood. Through the process of re-experiencing life circumstances and interactions with the analyst, the client becomes both intellectually and emotionally aware of the underlying source of current difficulties. However, this form of therapy is costly because it is inherently lengthy. Clients have traditionally paid their analyst directly for psychotherapeutic services, although in recent years some insurance plans have included coverage for psychological treatment, including psychoanalysis. Psychoanalysis is effective in treating a variety of mental disorders.

92. **Answer: 3**.

Cognitive-behavioral therapy is self-oriented. The therapist is a coach or teacher who helps the client learn how to manage his or her own life. The client learns new tools for living life and dealing with life's challenges. Cognitive therapy is considered task oriented, because interventions include homework assignments between sessions. For example, a client dealing with problems of anger and risk for violence may be asked to keep a journal detailing feelings of anger, situations bringing on angry feelings, and immediate behaviors following angry feelings. This has been highly successful in treating problems in which the client is intellectually intact. The client must be oriented in all three spheres and have the ability to complete homework assignments. It is inappropriate to conduct cognitive-behavioral therapy with one who is psychotic, demented, or unable or unwilling to cooperate actively with the therapist.

93. **Answer: 3**.

In the family-as-system approach, the family is viewed as more than the sum of its individual parts. Significant events that affect one family member also affect all other family members. Systems theory suggests that the individuals within a family are emotionally connected in such a way that any important event that affects one family member will have an effect on others as well. According to systems theory, when people are connected to each other in some meaningful way, events will necessitate a change or adjustment in all other parts of the system.

94. **Answer: 2**.

The trifocal model refers to wellness, prevention, and problem interventions. This model focuses on each nursing diagnosis individually.

95. **Answer: 4**.

When a nursing diagnosis of Caregiver Role Strain has been established, it is important for the nurse to include the caregiver in the health care planning team. This allows the caregiver to share concerns and actively explore alternative solutions to problems.

96. **Answer: 3**.

Ecomaps assist the nurse in understanding family dynamics. Ecomaps are a visual image of the interactions of all family members with systems outside of the family. These systems might include churches, community organizations, schools, and jobs.

97. **Answer: 2**.

The concept of universality is where a client learns that he or she is not alone and other people have the same or similar needs and difficulties. Clients may benefit by listening to the questions and concerns raised by other group members.

98. **Answer: 2**.

Capitation is best defined as a funding mechanism in which all defined services for a specified time are provided for an agreed-upon single payment. The payment is tied to the care of a particular client or group of clients. The provider contracts in advance to accept the risk for costs exceeding the agreed-on amount.

99. **Answer: 1**.

Relaxation techniques and guided imagery are examples of treatment modalities that are complementary, or adjunct, to other psychiatric treatment modalities. Relaxation is defined as a psychophysiological state characterized by parasympathetic dominance involving multiple visceral and somatic symptoms. Relaxation can reduce physical, mental, and emotional tension. Guided imagery involves visualizing sights, sounds, taste, touch, and smells. When the imagery is guided, the practitioner is the guide. Other forms of imagery can be initiated and controlled by the individual at his own discretion.

100. **Answer:** 4.

Centering involves focusing on one's self through activities such as relaxation imagery or praying for guidance. Once learned, this process takes only 30 to 60 seconds to perform and allows the nurse to re-energize self in order to address client needs. By centering, the nurse can be fully present with the client. The nurse is no longer distracted by the tensions in the environment.

NOTES

NOTES

NOTES

NOTES

NOTES

NOTES

NOTES

NOTES

NOTES

NOTES